Mental Health and Wellbeing:

A guide for nurses and allied healthcare professionals working with adults in primary care

Sheila Hardy

Mental Health and Wellbeing:

A guide for nurses and allied healthcare professionals working with adults in primary care

Sheila Hardy on behalf of the Charlie Waller Trust

M&K Publishing 2021

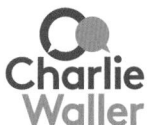

Full the full range of M&K Publishing books please visit our website:
www.mkupdate.co.uk

Mental Health and Wellbeing:
A guide for nurses and healthcare professionals working with adults in primary care
Sheila Hardy

ISBN: 978-1- 910451-14-4

First published 2021

British Library Catalogue in Publication Data
A catalogue record for this book is available from the British Library

Notice
Clinical practice and medical knowledge constantly evolve. Standard safety precautions must be followed, but, as knowledge is broadened by research, changes in practice, treatment and drug therapy may become necessary or appropriate. Readers must check the most current product information provided by the manufacturer of each drug to be administered and verify the dosages and correct administration, as well as contraindications. It is the responsibility of the practitioner, utilising the experience and knowledge of the patient, to determine dosages and the best treatment for each individual patient. Any brands mentioned in this book are as examples only and are not endorsed by the Publisher. Neither the publisher nor the authors assume any liability for any injury and/or damage to persons or property arising from this publication.

Disclaimer
M&K Publishing cannot accept responsibility for the contents of any linked website or online resource. The existence of a link does not imply any endorsement or recommendation of the organisation or the information or views which may be expressed in any linked website or online resource. We cannot guarantee that these links will operate consistently and we have no control over the availability of linked pages.

Printed by Bell & Bain Ltd, Glasgow
Typeset by Jeremy Fisher – www.processcreative.co.uk

The Publisher
To contact M&K Publishing write to:
M&K Update Ltd · The Old Bakery · St. John's Street
Keswick · Cumbria CA12 5AS
Tel: 01768 773030 · Fax: 01768 781099
publishing@mkupdate.co.uk
www.mkupdate.co.uk

Contents

Foreword

Nurses and allied health professionals are at the very heart of healthcare and will increasingly play a role in improving and even creating health. This book is an invaluable guide for people working with adults in primary care and will help them understand the different aspects of health and wellbeing and learn how to respond to the different conditions and situations they will be faced with. It is practical and to the point.

The Covid-19 pandemic has highlighted inequalities in our society and forced many people to think about health differently and in a wider, more holistic fashion. The World Health Organization (WHO) defines health as being about physical, mental and social wellbeing and Covid has shown us how important all three of these dimensions are. It is time now for us to give mental and social wellbeing much higher priority.

Worries about the health of ourselves and our families and friends, anxieties about employment, finances and the future, coupled with the constraints and loneliness of lockdown, have all affected our overall health for the worse. More positively, the pandemic has revealed the links between the health of individuals, the health of their communities, the health of society more generally and, ultimately, the health of the planet.

The pandemic is not, of course, the only driver of change. There has been a long-term shift in the burden of disease in recent years, with an enormous increase in the number of people with long-term or chronic conditions. This is in turn shifting ideas and practices in health and healthcare. Individuals take much more responsibility for their own health and wellbeing, many managing their conditions and making their own choices about what matters to them. Communities, social activities and relationships all have their part to play.

This has meant big changes for many health professionals, with a new emphasis on enabling, supporting and informing their patients (as expert guides and facilitators), alongside their role in specific interventions and treatments. A bio-psycho-social way of looking at their practice is replacing the focus on the medical model. Policy is changing too, albeit slowly, with a recognition that the solutions to most health issues lie in primary care and in the community, the places where people live, work and go to school. Health professionals working in these areas have a particular opportunity and responsibility to create the new services and practices that are needed for the future.

This book is a vital part of their preparation. It contains insights and wisdom drawn from many years of experience and is rich in practical advice and information. I am delighted to recommend it both to health professionals and to a wider audience.

Lord Nigel Crisp – Chief Executive of the NHS in England and Permanent Secretary of the UK Department of Health 2000–2006

About the author

Sheila Hardy PhD MSc BSc NISP RMN RGN
Practice Nurse Educator, Charlie Waller Trust

Sheila is a registered general and mental nurse with 20 years' clinical experience in primary care. Her PhD research involved training primary care health professionals to consider the physical health needs of people with severe mental illness.

In her role as trainer for the Charlie Waller Trust, Sheila develops and delivers mental health and wellbeing training to nurses and allied health care professionals in primary care, as well as mentoring nurses undertaking specific projects. Sheila has also worked for universities, a foundation trust, and an academic health science network. She enjoys educating others through training, research and writing articles and books.

Sheila has sat on several national expert reference and steering groups. In 2018 she won an Award of Merit from the Royal College of Nursing for her work on the physical health of people with mental illness.

The Charlie Waller Trust

The vision of the Charlie Waller Trust is of a world where people understand and talk openly about mental health, where young people and those who support them are equipped to maintain and enhance their mental health and wellbeing and have the confidence to seek help when they need it.

The Charlie Waller Trust was created by the Waller family in 1997, in response to the loss to suicide of their son and brother Charlie, who suffered from depression. They have since become one of the UK's most respected mental health charities.

Their overarching mission is to educate young people, and those with responsibility for them (including parents and carers, teachers, college and university staff, employers, GPs and Practice Nurses), about their mental health and wellbeing.

The focus of the Charlie Waller Trust is on supporting all young people, throughout their journey from primary school age to the early years of their working lives, recognising that the points of transition in that journey can represent moments of particular vulnerability.

They aim to improve young people's understanding of their own mental health, to give them the knowledge and skills to look out for and support themselves and those around them, and to give them greater confidence in talking openly about the subject. By enabling more open and better-informed conversations, they aim to further reduce the stigma that still surrounds mental health.

Most of the work undertaken by the Charlie Waller Trust is delivered through schools, parents, colleges and universities, and workplaces, in the form of consultancy, training, and the provision of educational and practical resources. They seek to establish enduring partnerships with such organisations, in order to bring about sustained change and lasting improvement.

This being their focus, they do not offer direct one-to-one support or advice for individuals. However, through their sponsorship of the Charlie Waller Institute at the University of Reading, they facilitate the training of clinicians in evidence-based psychological treatments, and associated research, so helping to increase the availability of expert help to individuals when they need it.

Overall, their approach is:
- **Positive** – focusing on prevention and early intervention and recognising the importance of offering hope
- **Proven** – their consultancy, training and resources are all based on sound clinical evidence
- **Practical** – their content provides people with strategies and tools to care for their mental health, and to support others in doing so.

The cornerstone of the Charlie Waller Trust's philosophy is that their training should be free at the point of need – this has been a key element of their approach since the charity's inception in 1997. They are not directly funded by Local Authorities or Clinical Commissioning Groups, so the majority of their work is enabled through fundraising.

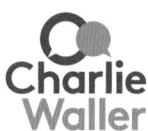

Introduction

Primary care is the first place people go to for healthcare advice and support. It is thought that one in three people attending primary care have a mental health problem. They do not always discuss their mental health issues with primary care staff but may voice other concerns linked to their mental health, such as physical symptoms or social concerns. Consequently, they may attend repeatedly before their underlying mental health problem is recognised.

People with long-term physical conditions, such as diabetes, are more likely to have mental health issues and will be healthier if both their physical and mental health are considered. Those with severe mental illness and a learning disability are more likely to die early from a physical cause than the rest of the population and this group therefore needs proactive monitoring and encouragement to promote healthy behaviour. People with dementia and their carers need support to live well; and those who are addicted to substances or specific behaviours need help to manage their dependence.

Most mental health support is provided by GPs, nurses and allied healthcare professionals working in primary care, where there is the opportunity to employ a holistic ('whole person') approach. However, many nurses and allied healthcare professionals have not undertaken any formal training in mental health. The Charlie Waller Trust (CWT) provides training for healthcare professionals in primary care, to help them meet the holistic needs of the people they see in healthcare settings every day. This book serves as a manual to accompany the training and as a learning resource in its own right.

I have written this book because my experience of training healthcare professionals has taught me how much they value written material which can be read at any time, whether or not they have access to a computer. I would like to thank CWT for supporting me to do this and I urge all readers of this book to visit the CWT website (https://charliewaller.org) to find out more about the fantastic work they do.

Sheila Hardy

CHAPTER 1

Promoting wellbeing

Learning outcomes

By the end of this chapter the reader will:

- Understand the factors which contribute to wellbeing
- Know how wellbeing can be measured
- Be aware of the steps to maintain wellbeing
- Understand how stress and distress can affect wellbeing
- Recognise stress and distress
- Be able to proactively help people to maintain their wellbeing

Introduction

Terms used when talking about wellbeing include: being in good health, health, wellness, healthiness, robustness and soundness. The World Health Organization (WHO) defines health as 'a state of complete physical, mental, and social wellbeing and not merely the absence of disease or infirmity' (WHO 2020). This definition has not been updated since 1948 and is sometimes criticised as being no longer fit for purpose and inadvertently promoting the medicalisation of society (Bickenbach 2015).

With the increase in the incidence of chronic disease, it has been proposed that more emphasis should be placed on having the ability to adapt and self-manage in the face of social, physical and emotional challenges (Huber, Knottnerus, *et al.* 2011).

What is wellbeing?

Wellbeing is about feeling good and functioning well. It encompasses a person's experience of their life, as well as their circumstances – compared with social standards and ideals. Wellbeing can be both subjective and objective.

Subjective wellbeing

Subjective wellbeing, sometimes referred to as personal wellbeing, means how people think and feel about their own wellbeing, and it includes:

- Life satisfaction (evaluation)
- Positive emotions (hedonic)
- Whether life is meaningful (eudaemonic).

Subjective wellbeing is measured by asking the person directly how they are feeling.

Objective wellbeing

Objective wellbeing is based on assumptions about basic human needs and rights, including:

- Adequate food
- Physical health
- Education
- Safety.

Objective wellbeing can be measured by asking people direct questions, or through more objective measures such as mortality rates and life expectancy.

The factors which contribute to wellbeing

The National Wellness Institute (Hettler 2018) cultivates a model of wellness that stresses the need for people to be proactive in enhancing and maintaining their health. It includes six dimensions of health: social, intellectual, emotional, occupational, spiritual, and physical. Environmental health is regularly added to these by other academics to make a list of seven dimensions.

Social

The social dimension involves relating to and connecting with other people. It includes establishing and maintaining positive relationships with family, friends and work colleagues.

It does not simply refer to being alone; it means being without some definite needed relationship or set of relationships and therefore experiencing loneliness (Mushtaq, Shoib, *et al.* 2014).

Social support increases resilience and promotes recovery from illness (Pevalin & Rose 2003). Resilience is a person's capacity to handle pressure and bounce back from adversity or their ability to persist and adjust when faced with challenges (Rutter 2008). Lack of social networks can affect mortality in the same way as clinical risks such as smoking, excessive alcohol consumption, obesity, raised cholesterol and hypertension (Pantell, Rehkopf *et al.* 2013) and can lead to mental and physical health problems (Mushtaq, Shoib, *et al.* 2014).

Conversely, having a mental health problem can increase the chances of feeling lonely (Mind 2019). It is more difficult to be happy if one compares oneself to others and focuses on one's weaknesses.

Wellbeing is improved when a person accepts themselves as they are; they can then be kinder to themselves when things go wrong.

Intellectual

The intellectual dimension includes the development of new skills, consideration of innovative ideas and experiences, and the application of learning to everyday life. Learning gives direction to people's lives (Teaching and Learning Research Programme 2008). It reduces the risk of developing depression and can lead to increased self-confidence, optimism and self-esteem (Tett & Maclachlan 2007). Choosing ambitious but realistic goals gives people a sense of direction and brings a sense of accomplishment and satisfaction when they achieve them.

Emotional

The emotional dimension refers to having an understanding of oneself, the ability to cope with life's challenges, and being able to acknowledge and share feelings in a productive manner.

Regularly experiencing positive emotions helps a person cope in difficult situations, as does focusing on the good aspects of a situation. Several experts agree that humans have four basic emotions: fear, anger, joy and sadness (Gu, Wang, *et al.* 2019). However, there is some disagreement among specialists as to the number of basic emotions, and proposed numbers range from two to eleven (Ortony & Turner 1990).

Table 1.1: Deeper emotions categorised using a short tree structure

Primary emotion	Secondary emotion	Tertiary emotions
Love	Affection	Adoration, affection, love, fondness, liking, attraction, caring, tenderness, compassion, sentimentality
	Lust	Arousal, desire, lust, passion, infatuation
	Longing	Longing
Joy	Cheerfulness	Amusement, bliss, cheerfulness, gaiety, glee, jolliness, joviality, joy, delight, enjoyment, gladness, happiness, jubilation, elation, satisfaction, ecstasy, euphoria
	Zest	Enthusiasm, zeal, zest, excitement, thrill, exhilaration
	Contentment	Contentment, pleasure
	Pride	Pride, triumph

Table continues overleaf

Primary emotion	Secondary emotion	Tertiary emotions
Joy	Optimism	Eagerness, hope, optimism
	Enthralment	Enthralment, rapture
	Relief	Relief
Surprise	Surprise	Amazement, surprise, astonishment
Anger	Irritation	Aggravation, irritation, agitation, annoyance, grouchiness, grumpiness
	Exasperation	Exasperation, frustration
	Rage	Anger, rage, outrage, fury, wrath, hostility, ferocity, bitterness, hate, loathing, scorn, spite, vengefulness, dislike, resentment
	Disgust	Disgust, revulsion, contempt
	Envy	Envy, jealousy
	Torment	Torment
Sadness	Suffering	Agony, suffering, hurt, anguish
	Sadness	Depression, despair, hopelessness, gloom, glumness, sadness, unhappiness, grief, sorrow, woe, misery, melancholy
	Disappointment	Dismay, disappointment, displeasure
	Shame	Guilt, shame, regret, remorse
	Neglect	Alienation, isolation, neglect, loneliness, rejection, homesickness, defeat, dejection, insecurity, embarrassment, humiliation, insult
	Sympathy	Pity, sympathy
Fear	Horror	Alarm, shock, fear, fright, horror, terror, panic, hysteria, mortification
	Nervousness	Anxiety, nervousness, tenseness, uneasiness, apprehension, worry, distress, dread

Adapted from Shaver, Schwartz, *et al.* (2001)

Occupational

The occupational dimension is the capacity to get personal satisfaction from work (or some other meaningful activity) while maintaining a positive work/life balance. Wellbeing is achieved through people's meaningful participation in daily life (Pollard, Kronenberg, *et al.* 2009). A lack of occupational opportunity has been associated with lower subjective experiences of wellbeing (Nilsson & Townsend 2010). People often arrange their occupational lives following a pattern or routine to give themselves a sense of value and community (Doble & Santha 2008).

Spiritual

The spiritual dimension refers to recognising meaning and purpose in life. It involves living consistently with one's values and opinions and being tolerant of the beliefs of others. It refers to the way individuals experience their connectedness to the moment, to self, to others, to nature, and to the significant or sacred (Pulchaski, Ferrell, *et al.* 2009). Spirituality does not have to be tied to any particular religious belief or tradition (Ellsworth & Ellsworth 2010). People's spiritual views and practices can affect the way they understand health and the strategies they use to cope with illness. They can also affect their resilience, resourcefulness and sense of support and their overall health outcomes (Hilbers, Haynes, *et al.* 2007).

Physical

The physical dimension is the ability to maintain a healthy quality of life by avoiding excessive fatigue or physical stress, and recognising which behaviours have an impact on wellness. As physical health is the most obvious dimension of health, it tends to be the most frequently used index to assess the wellbeing of individuals (Cho, Martin, *et al.* 2011). In terms of wellbeing, people in England (surveyed in 2013) consider physical health to be the most important aspect (Office for National Statistics (ONS) 2019).

Environmental

The environmental dimension means acknowledging responsibility for the quality of the surroundings or conditions in which a person lives or works, and the way these conditions influence how they feel and how effectively they can work. The wider determinants of environmental health include food safety, housing standards, health and safety, air quality, noise, and environment issues generally (DoH 2020).

According to the Department of Health (DoH 2014), the benefits of public wellbeing are:
- Years added to life
- Improved recovery from illness
- Positive health behaviours in adults and children
- Enhanced wellbeing and mental health of close family and friends
- Staff and healthcare providers work more effectively
- Better-quality decisions about patient care practice, treatment and costs
- Clearer decisions about local services
- Reduced healthcare burden.

Measuring wellbeing

A number of tools are used to measure wellbeing. Two are described here, the self-assessment tool used by the Office for National Statistics and the Warwick-Edinburgh Mental Wellbeing Scale.

Measuring wellbeing using a self-assessment tool

The Office for National Statistics (ONS) monitors personal wellbeing in the UK with an annual population survey (APS). Since April 2011, the tool they have included in the APS to do this consists of four questions:

1. Overall, how satisfied are you with your life nowadays?
2. Overall, to what extent do you feel the things you do in your life are worthwhile?
3. Overall, how happy did you feel yesterday?
4. Overall, how anxious did you feel yesterday?

Responses are given on a scale of 0 to 10, where 0 is 'not at all' and 10 is 'completely'. The ONS argues that these questions enable people to assess their lives overall, as well as providing an indication of their day-to-day emotions. Although 'yesterday' may not have been a typical day for every individual, the large sample surveyed means that these differences average out to give a reliable assessment of the anxiety and happiness of the adult population in the UK over the year.

Higher levels of personal wellbeing for life satisfaction, worth and happiness (questions 1–3) are defined as 7 or more out of 10. However, for anxiety (question 4), 3 or less out of 10 is a desirable score – because lower levels of anxiety indicate better personal wellbeing.

Key findings from the ONS Annual Population Survey

These are two of the headline results from April 2019 to March 2020 (ONS 2020):

- In the year ending March 2020, average ratings of life satisfaction, happiness and anxiety in the UK, all deteriorated. This was the first time since they started measuring them (in 2011) that these three measures have significantly worsened when compared with the year before.
- In the UK, average ratings of anxiety increased by 6.3% in the year ending March 2020 when compared with the year before, from 2.87 to 3.05 (out of 10); this was the largest annual increase in anxiety since the ONS began measuring personal wellbeing.

The Warwick-Edinburgh Mental Wellbeing Scale

There is no current guidance on measuring the wellbeing of people seen in primary care but there are tools which are relevant. The Warwick-Edinburgh Mental Wellbeing Scale or WEMWBS (Tennant, Hiller, *et al.* 2007) is often used by scientists and psychologists to measure wellbeing. There is also a shorter seven-question version (SWEMWBS). Both versions are free to use but are copyrighted by NHS Health Scotland and the Universities of Warwick and Edinburgh. To make use of them, you need to register on their website: https://warwick.ac.uk/fac/sci/med/research/platform/wemwbs/using

To get a person's wellbeing score, ask them to go through the statements and tick the box that best describes their thoughts and feelings over the last two weeks.

Statements	None of the time	Rarely	Some of the time	Often	All of the time
I've been feeling optimistic about the future	1	2	3	4	5
I've been feeling useful	1	2	3	4	5
I've been feeling relaxed	1	2	3	4	5
I've been feeling interested in other people	1	2	3	4	5
I've had energy to spare	1	2	3	4	5
I've been dealing with problems well	1	2	3	4	5
I've been thinking clearly	1	2	3	4	5
I've been feeling good about myself	1	2	3	4	5
I've been feeling close to other people	1	2	3	4	5
I've been feeling confident	1	2	3	4	5
I've been able to make up my own mind about things	1	2	3	4	5
I've been feeling loved	1	2	3	4	5
I've been interested in new things	1	2	3	4	5
I've been feeling cheerful	1	2	3	4	5

Then add up their total score.

If you explain that most people have a score between 41 and 59, this will help them to gauge what their score means.

If they have scored 0–40, ask the person if they would like some help to address their lack of mental wellbeing.

If they have scored 41–49, give positive feedback and advise the person that they can still improve their mental wellbeing by taking action.

If they have scored 59–70, give positive feedback and advise the person that they should continue doing the things that are keeping them well.

Steps to maintain wellbeing

The Foresight Mental Capital and Wellbeing Project was commissioned by the government in 2008 to independently review the evidence and consider the factors that influence an individual's mental development and wellbeing, from conception until death. The authors of this project have identified five steps, the wellbeing equivalent of 'five fruit and vegetables a day'.

Based on an extensive review of the evidence, the suggested actions are: Connect, Be active, Take notice, Keep learning, Give. These actions form the first five of the 'Ten Keys to Happier Living' (Action for Happiness 2020). These first five keys (GREAT) are about the way people interact with the **outside** world in their daily activities:

1. **G**iving – do things for others
2. **R**elating – connect with people
3. **E**xercising – take care of your body
4. **A**wareness – live life mindfully
5. **T**rying out – keep learning new things.

The second five keys (DREAM) come from **inside** the person and depend on their attitude to life:

6. **D**irection – Have goals to look forward to
7. **R**esilience – Find ways to bounce back
8. **E**motion – Take a positive approach
9. **A**cceptance – Be comfortable with who you are
10. **M**eaning – Be part of something bigger.

How stress can affect wellbeing

Initially, increased stress produces increased performance. But once the person passes a certain point, any more stress results in decreased performance. At this point, trying harder is therefore unproductive or even counterproductive. The only sensible thing to do is to take a break.

People need a certain amount of stress to function well, sometimes called healthy tension or eustress (good stress). However, stress becomes harmful (distress) when there is too much, when it lasts too long or when it occurs too often. One of the first symptoms of distress is fatigue, which is often ignored. If a person reports fatigue, then they should be advised to do something about it before it becomes exhaustion.

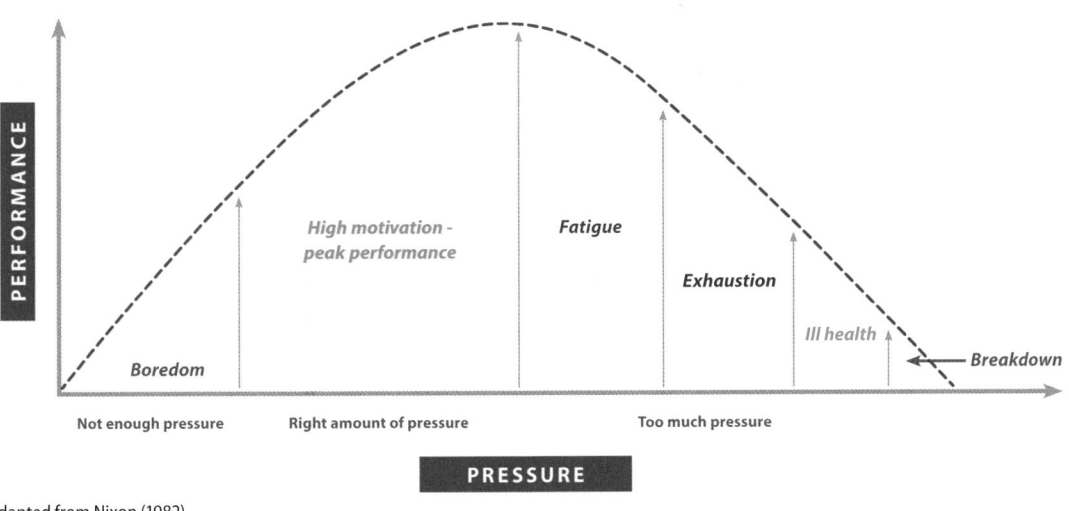

Adapted from Nixon (1982).

Figure 1.1 The effects of stress

Signs and symptoms

There are several signs and symptoms of stress that people may report. These can be divided into feelings, thoughts, behaviour, and physical symptoms.

Feelings:
- Moodiness
- Irritability or short temper
- Agitation, inability to relax
- Feeling overwhelmed
- Sense of loneliness and isolation
- General unhappiness.

Thoughts:
- Memory problems
- Inability to concentrate
- Poor judgement
- Seeing only the negative
- Anxious or racing thoughts
- Constant worrying.

Behaviour:

- Eating more or less
- Sleeping too much or too little
- Withdrawal
- Procrastinating or neglecting responsibilities
- Use of alcohol, cigarettes or drugs for relaxation
- Nervous habits (e.g. nail-biting, pacing).

Physical:

- Aches and pains
- Diarrhoea or constipation
- Nausea, dizziness
- Chest pain, rapid heartbeat
- Loss of libido
- Frequent colds.

Questions which may pick up symptoms of stress

If you suspect that someone is suffering from stress, asking the following questions may help to identify it:

- Are you able to sleep properly without any worries going through your mind?
- Do you feel impatient or irritable when confronted with minor problems?
- Do you find it difficult to concentrate because you are worrying about things?
- Are you finding it difficult to make decisions?
- Are you drinking or smoking more?
- Are you not enjoying food so much?
- Do you feel unable to relax because you feel that something always needs to be done?
- Do you feel tense, nauseous or sweaty?
- Do you feel that you have a 'knot' in your stomach, a dry mouth or a thumping heart?

If the person answers 'yes' to several of these questions, a gentle enquiry about the possible cause of stress may help them make a plan to alleviate it.

How distress can affect wellbeing

Distress is a feeling of extreme worry, sadness or pain. Many people living with physical conditions are distressed without being mentally ill, and their distress can lead to a poor quality of life.

They may not disclose problems to you without prompting, for several reasons, which may include:

- Not seeing problem-solving as the role of a healthcare professional
- Not expecting the healthcare professional to bring up the subject

- Feeling forced to 'think positively' by social pressure
- Lacking the social skills, confidence or verbal ability to disclose their problems
- Seeing the healthcare professional as too busy
- Feeling too ashamed to admit they have certain problems
- Thinking that they will be seen as complaining, ungrateful or a nuisance
- Feeling guilty, for example, about their lifestyle
- Thinking the distress is an expected part of their condition
- Worrying that they will be viewed as mentally ill or unable to cope.

Screening for distress

The King's Fund (2012) recommends making use of consultation techniques that normalise the discussion of mental and emotional aspects of physical illness. Using a tool can help the person to identify particular areas of difficulty. They can then work with the healthcare professional to look at the best way to tackle their problems.

The Distress Thermometer is a tool which can be used to screen people for distress from any source (Roth, Kornblith, *et al.* 1998). It was originally developed for use in people with cancer and is recommended by the National Institute for Health and Care Excellence (NICE) for people with language difficulties or sensory impairment (NICE 2009). Research has been carried out to show that it can be useful in managing long-term conditions such as stroke (Gillespie & Cadden 2013). This tool can enhance communication between patients and healthcare professionals as it allows a range of anxieties to be explored. It can be downloaded from the NCCN website. The tool contains a picture of a thermometer on one side which depicts no distress as a score of zero and extreme distress as a score of 10. On the other side it has a list of problems under the headings of practical, family, emotional and physical, and a space for anything else which does not fit under the headings.

NCCN have provided the following written guidance for its use.

How to use the Distress Thermometer

It is preferable that the person is alone so that they feel comfortable discussing their anxieties. However, there are times when this is not possible – for example, if they have special needs or require an interpreter, or they want a friend or relative to be present.

Introducing the patient to the Distress Thermometer:

- Ask the person if they are happy to be asked some questions to see how their condition is affecting them, using an assessment form.
- Show them the form. If they say they don't want to do it, reassure them that's OK. Gently ask if they would mind telling you why they don't want to complete it.

Completing the Distress Thermometer:

- Show the person the picture of the Distress Thermometer. Ask whether they have felt distressed during the past week; then choose a number on the thermometer that signifies how distressed they have been over the past week, including today. Ask them to circle the number (0–10). If they have not been distressed at all, they should circle 0. If they score 4 or above, they are considered to be distressed (Mitchell 2007).
- Then show them the Problem List. If any of the items listed have been a cause of distress for them over the past week, including today, ask them to tick the box next to it (leave it blank if it does not apply).
- Explain that if there is something causing them distress that is not on the list, they can add it.
- Where multiple items of distress are identified, ask which one is bothering them the most and focus on this one. Others can be dealt with in order of priority later.
- Ask open questions to find out more about the main problem. This is an opportunity for the person to tell you about their feelings and experiences. Often, they can be reassured that these are normal.
- Keep the discussion positive:
  - o Highlight times where the person has managed well and build on these positive examples.
  - o Focus on solutions, rather than the difficulties encountered.

Helping people to maintain their wellbeing

People can be assisted to maintain their wellbeing through an organisational approach and during consultations.

Using an organisational approach to maintain wellbeing

Some examples of using an organisational approach to maintain wellbeing are given below.

What a GP practice can do to promote wellbeing:

1. **Provide relevant up-to-date information (to empower individuals), using:**
- Appropriate leaflets
- Poster displays
- Feature on website
- Signposting to other resources
- Long-term condition clinics designed to promote self-management.

2. **Allow prompt access to an appropriate healthcare professional (to reduce anxiety, and prevent symptoms worsening) by:**
- Phone
- Email
- Consultation.

3. **Find out what the patient population want (to give patients a sense of ownership) through:**
● Patient participation groups
● Surveys designed by patients.

4. **Provide group support (to connect with others and give to others) with:**
● Education groups (e.g. for particular conditions, health promotion, wellbeing)
● Carers' groups
● Smoking cessation groups
● Signposting to third sector agencies.

5. **Promote activity through:**
● Exercise on referral
● Walking groups
● Access to physiotherapy.

6. **Consider the patients' experience (prevents frustration, increases trust):**
● If appointments are always running late, schedule more time for each one (so that patients won't have to wait)
● Consider the wellbeing of the staff
● Educate all staff in mental health awareness
● Educate all clinical staff to understand how to promote wellbeing and care for people with specific mental health problems.

Get leaflets/posters for your practice: www.actionforhappiness.org/poster-great-dream

Using consultations to maintain wellbeing

Helping people learn how to maintain their wellbeing can be preventative (if they already have good wellbeing) or restorative (if they are experiencing or recovering from stress, distress, depression or anxiety).

Healthcare professionals may notice that a person is behaving in a manner that could be detrimental to their wellbeing, but they need to seek permission to offer assistance. While the healthcare professional may see the obvious benefits of making changes to their lifestyle, the person may not be so convinced. This is why it is vital to develop skills in recognising the person's readiness to change and responding appropriately.

Healthcare professionals can use consultations to maintain wellbeing by promoting healthy lifestyle habits, including checking caffeine intake, encouraging healthy eating, promoting regular exercise, advising on sleep hygiene, and giving support with addictions (for more on all this, see Chapter 2). They can also teach people how to do self-help exercises.

Self-help exercises

Worry time

Set time aside each day to deal with your worries. Half an hour is usually adequate. People tend to get better at doing this, the more they practise. There are two aspects: planning how to deal with your worries; and identifying your worries.

Planning how to deal with worries:

1. Make a list of the tasks that need to be dealt with the next day.

2. Timetable the tasks into the day.

3. Identify any areas where assistance may be required.

4. Identify the source of help needed and timetable this into the day.

Identifying worries:

1. Write down all your worries on a blank sheet of paper. Don't think about them, just list them.

2. Look through your list and put a line through any worries that are not really yours (e.g. two friends who are not getting on and this is worrying you). These are not your worries.

3. Choose one of your remaining worries and do one thing about that particular issue. Even if the step taken is a small one, something has been done, rather than just worrying.

4. Plan your next assigned worry time.

Relaxation

Relaxation can both prevent and relieve the symptoms of stress. Releasing any tension in the body and clearing thoughts helps the person to deal with any issues. When recommending any form of relaxation to people, it is important to explain that these skills need to be learned and they take practice. Many people give up before feeling the benefits because they cannot do it straight away. Ways to relax include relaxation exercises, meditation and mindfulness.

Two forms of relaxation exercises are described below: relaxed breathing and deep muscle relaxation.

Relaxed breathing

Practise deep breathing at a regular time and in a quiet place where you won't be disturbed. Loosen or remove any tight clothes, such as shoes or jackets. Be completely comfortable.

Sit in a comfortable chair which supports your head or lie on the floor or bed. Place your arms on the chair arms, or flat on the floor or bed, a little bit away from the sides of your body, with the palms up. If you're lying down, stretch out your legs, keeping them hip-width apart or slightly wider. If you're sitting in a chair, don't cross your legs.

Good relaxation always starts with focusing on your breathing:

- If you breathe in and out slowly and in a regular rhythm, this will help you to calm down.
- Fill up the whole of your lungs with air, without forcing. Imagine you're filling up a bottle, so that your lungs fill from the bottom.
- Breathe in through your nose and out through your mouth.
- Breathe in slowly and regularly, counting from one to five (don't worry if you can't reach five at first).
- Then let the breath escape slowly, counting from one to five.
- Keep doing this until you feel calm. Breathe without pausing or holding your breath.

Practise this relaxed breathing for 3 to 5 minutes, two to three times a day (or whenever you feel the need to calm down).

Deep muscle relaxation

This technique takes around 20 minutes. It flexes or stretches different muscles in turn and then relaxes them. This releases tension from the body and relaxes the mind.

Find a warm, quiet place with no distractions. Get completely comfortable, either sitting or lying down. Close your eyes and begin by focusing on your breathing. Breathe slowly and deeply, as described above.

If you have pain in certain muscles, or if there are muscles that you find it difficult to focus on, spend more time on relaxing other parts of your body.

For each exercise, hold the stretch for a few seconds, and then relax. Repeat a couple of times. Working through the muscle groups in the same order makes sure no part of the body is missed:

- Face: push your eyebrows together, as though frowning, then release.
- Neck: gently tilt the head forwards, pushing chin down towards chest, then slowly lift again.
- Shoulders: pull them up towards the ears (shrug), then relax them down towards the feet.
- Chest: breathe slowly and deeply into the diaphragm (below your bottom rib) so that you're using the whole of your lungs. Then breathe slowly out, allowing your belly to deflate as all the air is exhaled.
- Arms: stretch your arms away from your body, reach, then relax.
- Legs: push your toes away from your body, then pull them towards your body, then relax.
- Wrists and hands: stretch your wrist by pulling your hand up towards you, and stretch out the fingers and thumbs, then relax.

Spend some time lying (or sitting) quietly after your relaxation with your eyes closed. When you feel ready, stretch and get up slowly.

Meditation

The purpose of meditation is to focus and quiet the mind, eventually reaching a higher level of awareness and inner calm. Meditation can be done anywhere and at any time, allowing the person to access a sense of tranquillity and peace, no matter what is going on around them. Yoga is a form of meditation which is easily accessible.

Mindfulness

Mindfulness can help change the way a person thinks and feels about stress. It is a combination of meditation, breathing techniques and paying attention to the present moment. Ways to practise mindfulness include following everyday mindful practices, virtual applications, online courses and formal group courses.

Everyday mindful practices

Everyday mindful practice can be carried out in several ways. For instance:

- Pick a time, for example on your journey to work.
- Try new things, such as taking a different route or going somewhere new to buy groceries.
- Take notice of your thoughts and feelings. Silently naming them and letting them go can be helpful, e.g. 'Here is a thought that…' or 'This is anxiety'.
- Notice physical sensations, such as the taste of food, or the feel of wind in your hair or rain on your skin.
- Observe your own thoughts – stand back and watch them floating past, like leaves on a stream.

Mindfulness apps

There are mindfulness apps that can be downloaded onto a tablet or mobile phone. Here are some examples:

- Stop, Breathe & Think: https://www.stopbreathethink.com/about/
- Meditation for a happier, healthier you: https://www.tenpercent.com/
- Calm: www.calm.com
- The Mindfulness Training App: https://www.smilingmind.com.au/

Online mindfulness courses

Patients can sign up for an online course where they learn through self-directed practice at home. A free course is available, modelled on the MBSR program founded by Jon Kabat-Zinn at the University of Massachusetts. http://palousemindfulness.com/selfguidedMBSR.html

Formal group mindfulness courses

There may be courses commissioned in some areas for NHS patients; healthcare professionals should check with their local Clinical Commissioning Group (CCG).

Time outs and leisure

To remain well and prevent stress, people need breaks from work and time for themselves. It is a balance that people often get wrong because of outside pressure. People can be assisted to plan this balance using a behaviour diary. This can be a paper version or it may be on a device such as a tablet or mobile phone. The person plans all their activities for the week and it is most important that they schedule in 'relaxation' time. They then follow the plan!

Helping people to change stressful situations

Money management

Being in debt or worrying about how to manage one's finances can cause a great deal of stress. Healthcare professionals can help people by offering a listening ear, providing written information and signposting them to organisations who can provide practical advice, such as:

● National Debtline – http://www.nationaldebtline.co.uk/
● Step Change – http://www.stepchange.org/Howwecanhelpyou/Debtadvice.aspx
● Citizens' Advice Bureau – https://www.citizensadvice.org.uk/debt-and-money/help-with-debt/

Being assertive

Stress often arises when a person is unable to assert their opinion or view. This can lead to overwork, performing inappropriate tasks or being put in situations which they find uncomfortable. These circumstances can be in the home or the workplace. You can support the person by being a non-judgemental confidant. The options open to the person will depend on their situation. It is always advisable to try and sort the problem out directly with the person involved. If this is not possible, here are a few organisations that may be able to help:

● Advisory, Conciliation and Arbitration Service (ACAS – employment issues) – Helpline: 08457 47 47 47
   http://www.acas.org.uk/index.aspx?articleid=797
● Relate (relationship counselling) – https://www.relate.org.uk/
● Citizen's advice Bureau – http://www.citizensadvice.org.uk/index/getadvice.htm
● Links to information regarding assertiveness skills – http://www.moodjuice.scot.nhs.uk/Assertiveness.asp

Problem-solving

Providing an opportunity for people to talk about their problems is not only therapeutic but can help them to see things from a different point of view. This may open up potential solutions.

When facilitating problem-solving, the healthcare professional should methodically work through these key steps.

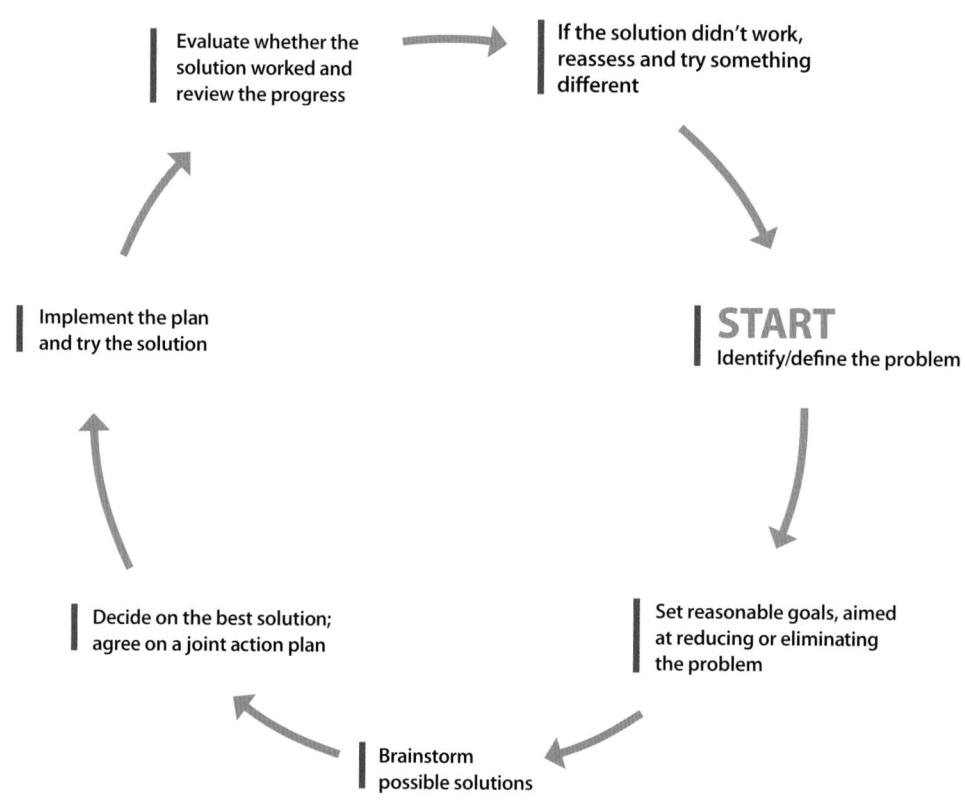

Figure 1.2 Key steps in problem-solving

Defining the problem

The following questions may be helpful in defining the person's problem:

1. How is your usual routine affected?

2. Does the problem only occur at a certain time or place?

3. Does the problem only occur when you are with a certain person or group of people?

4. Is the problem preventing you from doing anything?

Then:

- Discuss one problem at a time
- Divide one big problem into smaller problems
- Tackle problems one at a time
- Avoid vague problem definitions
- Define problems briefly.

Always finish one step thoroughly before you move onto the next step.

Helping the person to set a goal to make a positive change

The person should be encouraged to identify their goal which should be **S**pecific, **M**easurable, **A**chievable, **R**ealistic and **T**imely (**SMART**).

They can then list the possible solutions. Once solutions have been identified, their good points and bad points should be recorded as points 'for' and 'against'.

Solution	For	Against

They should then be asked which seems the best solution to the problem and then set a realistic target date to implement their chosen solution.

Solving the problem

The person may need help to decide on the steps needed to ensure that the chosen solution succeeds. It may be useful to involve others to help achieve it. Making a plan is helpful, using the following template.

Problem:	
Goal:	Target Date:
Plan:	
Progress:	

Helping people to change their thinking

Wellbeing is more likely to be maintained when people: look at things more positively; see problems as opportunities; refute negative thoughts; and keep a sense of humour. This does not come naturally to everyone but can be learnt.

Your local Improving Access to Psychological Therapies (IAPT) service may offer this service http://www.nhs.uk/Service-Search/Psychological%20therapies%20(IAPT)/LocationSearch/10008

Wellbeing plan

Some people may benefit from having their own 'wellbeing' plan. Discussing and reviewing this plan provides an opportunity to give support and encouragement. This is an example of a wellbeing plan, in which the right-hand column can be completed after discussion.

Things to do to stay well
Things to do every day
Things to do every week
Things to avoid
How other people can help me
Where I can go for help

Summary

Maintaining wellbeing has benefits for the individual and their family members and can reduce the burden on healthcare services. Healthcare professionals in primary care can help patients preserve and restore their wellbeing by using an organisational approach, and by promoting healthy lifestyles and teaching self-help exercises during consultations.

Vignette

Julie is 41 years old with two pre-teenage boys. She works full-time in a clothes shop. She is married to Dave who works away during the week. She has come to the primary care centre because she feels generally tired and full of aches and pains. She admits to increasing her alcohol intake and eating more.

How should the healthcare professional approach the consultation?

Reflective questions

- If a person was experiencing stress, what support would they receive from healthcare professionals in your primary care centre?
- What does your primary care centre currently provide to promote the wellbeing of staff and patients?
- How could your primary care centre demonstrate to patients the importance of improving and maintaining their physical and mental wellbeing?

References

Action for Happiness (2020). *10 Keys to Happier Living.* https://www.actionforhappiness.org/10-keys-to-happier-living (Last accessed 23.8.2021).

Bickenbach, J. (2015), WHO's definition of health: Philosophical analysis. In: T. Schramme & S. Edwards (eds) *Handbook of the Philosophy of Medicine.* Dordrecht: Springer.

Cho, J., Martin, P., Margrett, J. *et al.* (2011). The relationship between physical health and psychological well-being among oldest-old adults. *Journal of Aging Research.* **11** https://doi.org/10.4061/2011/605041 (Last accessed 23.8.2021).

Department of Health (DoH) (2014). *Wellbeing: Why it matters to health policy.* https://assets.publishing.service.gov.uk/government/uploads/system/uploads/attachment_data/file/277566/Narrative__January_2014_.pdf (Last accessed 23.8.2021).

Department of Health (DoH) (2020). *Environmental Health.* https://www.health-ni.gov.uk/topics/professional-medical-and-environmental-health-advice/environmental-health (Last accessed 23.8.2021).

Doble, S. & Santha, J. (2008). Occupational well-being: Rethinking occupational therapy outcomes. *Canadian Journal of Occupational Therapy.* **75** (3), 184–190.

Ellsworth, R. & Ellsworth J. (2010). Editorial: Special issue on spirituality, mental health and wellbeing. *International Journal of Applied Psychoanalytic Studies.* **7** (2). 99–101.

Foresight Mental Capital and Wellbeing Project (2008). *Final Project report – Executive summary.* London: The Government Office for Science.

Gillespie, D. & Cadden, P. (2013). The Distress Management System for Stroke (DMSS): An approach for screening and initial intervention for post-stroke psychological distress. *Journal of Nursing Education and Practice.* **3** (10). 150–158.

Gu, S., Wang, F., Patel, N. *et al.* (2019). A model for basic emotions using observations of behavior in Drosophila. *Frontiers in Psychology.* **10**, 781.

Hettler, B. (2018). The six dimensions of wellness. https://www.nationalwellness.org/page/Six_Dimensions (Last accessed 23.8.2021).

Hilbers, J., Haynes, A., Kivikko, J. *et al.* (2007). *Spirituality/Religion and Health Research report (phase two).* Sydney: SESIAHS 25.

Huber, M., Knottnerus, J., Green, L. *et al.* (2011). How should we define health? *British Medical Journal.* 343 d4163.

Mind (2019). *Loneliness.* https://www.mind.org.uk/media-a/3124/loneliness-2019.pdf (Last accessed 23.8.2021).

Mitchell, A. (2007). Pooled results from 38 analyses of the accuracy of the distress thermometer and other ultra-short methods of detecting cancer related mood disorders. *Journal of Clinical Oncology.* **25**, 4670–4681.

Mushtaq, R., Shoib, S., Shah, T. *et al.* (2014). Relationship between loneliness, psychiatric disorders and physical health? A review on the psychological aspects of loneliness. *Journal of Clinical and Diagnostic Research.* **8** (9) WE01–WE4.

National Institute for Health and Care Excellence (NICE) (2009). Depression in adults with a chronic physical health problem. https://www.nice.org.uk/Guidance/CG91 (Last accessed 23.8.2021).

Nilsson, I. & Townsend, E. (2010). Occupational justice – bridging theory and practice. *Scandinavian Journal of Occupational Therapy.* **17**, 57–63.

Nixon, P.G. (1982). The human function curve – a paradigm for our times. *Activitas Nervosa Superior* (Praha). Supplement 3(Pt 1), 130–133. PMID: 7183056.

Office for National Statistics (ONS) (2019). *Measuring national well-being in the UK: international comparisons.* https://www.ons.gov.uk/peoplepopulationandcommunity/wellbeing/articles/measuringnationalwellbeing/internationalcomparisons2019#health (Last accessed 23.8.2021).

Office for National Statistics (ONS) (2020). *Personal well-being in the UK: April 2019 to March 2020.* https://www.ons.gov.uk/peoplepopulationandcommunity/wellbeing/bulletins/measuringnationalwellbeing/april2019tomarch2020 (Last accessed 23.8.2021).

Ortony, A. & Turner, T. (1990), What's basic about basic emotions? *Psychological Review.* **97**, 315–331.

Pantell, M., Rehkopf, D., Jutt, D. *et al.* (2013). Social isolation: a predictor of mortality comparable to traditional clinical risk factors. *American Journal of Public Health.* **103** (11), 2056–2062.

Pevalin, D. & Rose, D. (2003). *Social Capital for Health: Investigating the links between social capital and health using the British Household Panel Survey.* Health Development Agency.

Pollard, N., Kronenberg, F. & Sakellariou, D. (2009). *A Political Practice of Occupational Therapy.* Edinburgh: Elsevier.

Pulchaski, C., Ferrell, B., Virani, R. *et al.* (2009). Improving the quality of spiritual care as a dimension of palliative care: The report of the consensus conference. *Journal of Palliative Medicine.* **12**, 886–904.

Roth, A., Kornblith, A., Batel-Copel, L. *et al.* (1998). Rapid screening for psychologic distress in men with prostate carcinoma: a pilot study. *Cancer.* **82**, 1904–1908.

Rutter, M. (2008). Developing concepts in developmental psychopathology, 3–22. In: J.J. Hudziak (ed.) *Developmental Psychopathology and Wellness: Genetic and Environmental Influences.* Washington, DC: American Psychiatric Publishing.

Shaver, P., Schwartz, J., Kirson, D. *et al.* (2001). Emotional knowledge: Further exploration of a prototype approach. In: G. Parrott (ed.), *Emotions in Social Psychology: Essential Readings.* 26–56. Philadelphia, PA: Psychology Press.

Teaching and Learning Research Programme (2008). *Learning Lives Research Briefing No. 51: Learning Lives: Learning, identity and agency in the life course.* London: Teaching and Learning Research Programme.

Tennant, R., Hiller, L., Fishwick, R., *et al.* (2007). The Warwick-Edinburgh Mental Wellbeing Scale (WEMWBS): Development and UK validation. *Health and Quality of Life Outcome.* **5**, 63. doi:101186/1477-7252-5-63)

Tett, L. & Maclachlan, K. (2007). Adult literacy and numeracy, social capital, learner identities and self-confidence. *Studies in the Education of Adults.* **39** (2), 150–167.

The King's Fund and Centre for Mental Health (2012). Long-term conditions and mental health: The cost of co-morbidities. http://www.kingsfund.org.uk/sites/files/kf/field/field_publication_file/long-term-conditions-mental-health-cost-comorbidities-naylor-feb12.pdf (Last accessed 23.8.2021).

World Health Organization (WHO) (2020). What is the WHO definition of health? https://www.who.int/about/frequently-asked-questions#:~:text=Health%20is%20a%20state%20of,absence%20of%20disease%20or%20infirmity. (Last accessed 23.8.2021).

CHAPTER 2

Encouraging healthy behaviour

Learning outcomes

By the end of this chapter the reader will:

- Be able to define behaviour
- Be aware of the lifestyle behaviours that keep people healthy
- Understand how to assess readiness to change behaviour
- Know how to respond to people at each stage of readiness
- Feel able to support people to change their behaviour using a structured approach

Introduction

Behaviour is usually defined as the observable and measurable actions displayed by a person. Healthy behaviour means activity undertaken by an individual for the purpose of maintaining or enhancing their health, preventing health problems, or achieving a positive body image (Cockerham 2014). The purpose of the behaviour can be described as the outcome, for example doing daily sit-ups (behaviour) to achieve a flatter stomach (outcome).

To understand how a behaviour is defined, do this short quiz (see answers at the end of this chapter).

Is this a behaviour?

a) Brushing your teeth

b) Losing weight

c) Jogging on the spot

d) Playing bingo

e) Lowering cholesterol

f) Having shiny hair

g) Eating crisps

Healthy lifestyle behaviours

Healthy lifestyle behaviours include eating healthily, exercising regularly, getting adequate rest and relaxation, limiting caffeine and alcohol intake, avoiding drugs and smoking, maintaining personal care, and seeking medical care when required (Eliopoulos 2010). Behavioural addictions can also have a detrimental effect on health (Alavi, Ferdosi, *et al.* 2012).

Healthy eating

Eating a healthy diet increases the chance of living longer and can help prevent some diseases (Mehta & Myrskyl 2017). Food plays an important role in the development, management and prevention of some mental health problems, such as depression (Clay 2017). A study showed that making small dietary changes, such as eating less junk food and more nutrient-rich foods, can make a big difference to depression (Jacka, O'Neil, *et al.* 2017). Wellbeing can be protected when the diet provides adequate nutrients (complex carbohydrates, essential fats, amino acids, vitamins and minerals and fluids) and avoids overindulgence in alcohol and unhealthy foods (Mental Health Foundation 2007).

There are many healthy eating websites available – here is a good example: https://www.nhs.uk/live-well/eat-well/

A 'food and mood' diary, which aims to help a person understand how the way they feel is affected by what they drink and eat, can be very helpful. The type of food is recorded in the diary, along with mood before and after.

Time	Type of food	Quantity	Mood before	Mood after

Examples of mood: happy, sad, angry, scared.

A sample 'food and mood' diary can be downloaded from this website:
http://www.personal-nutrition-guide.com/support-files/food_mood_journal.pdf

Regular exercise

Regular exercise increases a person's strength, flexibility and endurance (Ferreira, Sherrington, *et al.* 2012). It decreases the risk of coronary heart disease and stroke, diabetes, hypertension, osteoporosis, various types of cancer, and depression; and is essential to energy balance and weight control (WHO 2018).

Regular exercise also triggers the release of endorphins, which make the person feel good, and helps give structure and purpose to the day (Dfarhud, Malmir, *et al.* 2014, Hooker & Masters 2018). When the exercise is taken outdoors, exposure to sunlight affects the pineal gland and directly boosts mood (Pudikov & Dorokhov 2012). To stay healthy or improve health, adults need to do two types of physical activity each week: aerobic (to improve the efficiency of the body's cardiovascular system in absorbing and transporting oxygen); and anaerobic (building strength) exercises (NHS 2019). The key to a successful exercise regime is for the person to find something that they enjoy and can maintain.

Here are some examples:
- Walking can be built up as the person's fitness level increases. It can be done almost anywhere, at no cost.
- Swimming and cycling are good for people who find weight-bearing exercise difficult.
- Group exercise provides a way of meeting others and can help the person to maintain the activity. Park Run, rambling clubs and exercise classes all offer good opportunities to get fit with other people.

Rest and relaxation

Regular rest and relaxation, along with high-quality sleep, are necessary for the body to function normally. Adults should aim to have between seven and nine hours of sleep a night (Hirshkowitz, Whiton, *et al.* 2015). Certain activities take place during sleep, including removing waste material from the brain, restoration of bodily functions, repair of damaged tissues and conservation of energy (Kryger 2017). A lack of sleep leads to exaggerated sensitivity to pain, alters the immune response and the pattern of hormonal secretion (especially the growth hormone), and enhances the risk of obesity, diabetes, and cardiovascular disease (Orzeł-Gryglewska 2010). Perception, concentration, memory, vision, reactions, decision-making, and emotions can all be affected when sleep is poor (Orzeł-Gryglewska 2010). This increases the risk of road traffic accidents and can lead to low productivity and mistakes at work (Colten & Altevogt 2006). Too much sleep can also be detrimental to physical and mental health (Devore, Grodstein, *et al.* 2014).

The following good sleep habits, also known as sleep hygiene, can help people get a good night's sleep:
1. Maintain a regular routine. Going to bed and getting up at roughly the same time every day programs the body to sleep better.
2. Create a restful sleeping environment. The bedroom should be kept for rest and sleep. Temperature, lighting and noise should be controlled so that the bedroom environment helps the person to fall (and stay) asleep.
3. Have a comfortable bed. Sleep is difficult if the person is uncomfortable.

4. Take regular moderate exercise. This reduces tension and makes the body tired. However, vigorous exercise too close to bedtime should be avoided.

5. Avoid caffeine. Caffeine can affect the process of falling asleep and prevent deep sleep. A warm, milky drink is preferable in the evening. Herbal tea is also a good hot drink substitute for tea or coffee before bed.

6. Avoid over-indulgence. Too much food or alcohol (especially late at night) can interrupt sleep patterns. Alcohol may assist the person in getting to sleep initially, but it can disrupt sleep later.

7. Stop smoking. People who smoke take longer to fall asleep and also wake up more frequently.

8. Relax before bed. Some useful methods include: having a warm bath; listening to quiet music; doing some yoga or relaxation exercises.

9. Worry time. Deal with worries or a heavy workload by making lists of things to be tackled the next day. If you tend to lie in bed thinking about tomorrow's tasks, set aside time before bedtime to review the day and make plans for the next day. The goal is to avoid doing these things when you are in bed, trying to sleep.

10. Do not worry in bed. If you cannot sleep, do not lie there worrying about it. Get up and do something you find relaxing until you feel sleepy again, then return to bed

Caffeine

Caffeine stimulates the central nervous system. It is present in drinks such as coffee, tea and cola. It is also present in some chocolate. Too much caffeine can cause feelings of anxiety and nervousness, sleep disruption (especially difficulty getting off to sleep), restlessness, irritability, increased diuresis, stomach complaints, trembling, palpitations and arrhythmias. Experts agree that moderate daily caffeine intake, at dosages of up to 400mg a day, is not associated with adverse effects in healthy adults (Temple, Bernard, *et al.* 2017).

Caffeine Content

Item	Caffeine content (mg/100mL)	Serving size (mL)	Caffeine content (mg/serving)
Filter coffee	60–100	150	90–150
Instant coffee	27–72	150	40–108
Decaffeinated coffee	1–3	150	2–5
Weak tea	6–22	150	9–33
Strong tea	13–33	150	20–50
Cold (iced) tea	6–10	350	22–36
Hot cocoa	1–5	175	2–8

Item	Caffeine content (mg/100mL)	Serving size (mL)	Caffeine content (mg/serving)
Chocolate milk	1–3	235	2–7
Milk chocolate	3–50	30	1–15
Baking chocolate	115	30	35
Coca-Cola®	10	350	35
Diet Coke®	13	350	47
Pepsi®	11	350	38
Diet Pepsi®	10	350	36
Dr Pepper®	11	350	40
Red Bull®	34	235	80

Adapted from McLellan & Lieberman (2012), Lieberman, Carvey, et al. (2010)

Alcohol

The United Kingdom's Chief Medical Officer recommends limiting alcohol intake to under 14 units per week to avoid the risks associated with alcohol (DoH 2016). These risks include chronic health problems (mental health problems, liver, neurological, gastrointestinal and cardiovascular conditions and several types of cancer), and alcohol-related accidents, injuries and poisoning (Rehm, Baliunas, *et al.* 2010).

Drugs

Depending on the specific drug or drugs used, how they are taken, how much is taken, the person's health, and other factors, drugs have a wide range of short- and long-term effects (NIDA 2020). The short-term effects include appetite change, difficulty in sleeping, increased heart rate and blood pressure, overdose, changes in mood and psychosis. More serious consequences are myocardial infarction, stroke and death. The long-term effects include heart disease, lung disease, cancer, HIV/AIDS, hepatitis, mental illness and addiction.

There are also some indirect negative effects of drug use on both the person who is taking drugs and on those around them. These include risk for trauma, violence, injury and communicable diseases; negative effects on education, employment, housing, relationships; and increased risk of criminal activity (NIDA 2020).

Smoking

Smoking tobacco is associated with various cancers, lung and cardiovascular problems, osteoporosis, complications in pregnancy, infertility, oral health problems, and aging skin (NHS 2020). It can also affect learning and memory (Marshall, Heffernan, *et al.* 2016).

Medical self-care

Medical self-care can be described as the actions that a person takes to manage minor illness and injuries at home and to prevent, detect, and treat an illness or condition (DoH 2005). This includes seeking emergency and routine medical care as necessary, and behaviour that will assist in avoiding illness and injury such as safe sex, visiting the dentist/doctor when invited for screening, and being careful to avoid accidents.

Personal self-care

Personal self-care can be emotional, physical, social, practical, mental and spiritual (Planned Parenthood 2020).

- Emotional self-care involves activities that help the person connect, process and reflect on a full range of emotions – for example, keeping a journal, playing music, counselling.
- Physical self-care consists of activities that improve or protect physical health – for example, taking regular exercise, eating healthily, avoiding alcohol.
- Social self-care comprises actions that cultivate relationships – for example, eating out with friends, making time to telephone family regularly.
- Practical self-care includes tasks that prevent future stressful situations – for example, writing a shopping list, putting items away where they can be found, packing early.
- Mental self-care is taking part in an activity that stimulates the mind or intellect – for example, reading a book, doing a puzzle, going to a museum.
- Spiritual self-care involves activities that nurture the spirit and allow the person to think beyond themselves. This does not have to be religious – for or example, it could involve meditation, yoga, going to a place of worship, being in nature, or self-reflection.

Behavioural addictions

People can become addicted to almost any behaviour that gives them a strong sense of being rewarded (Addictions UK 2020). The addictions can involve normal behaviour, such as sex, eating, work and internet use; or gambling, which is recognised in psychiatric diagnosis (Petry, Zajac, *et al.* 2018). Behavioural addictions can result in problems in many areas of the individual's life (Alavi *et al.* 2012). Addictions are discussed more fully in Chapter 7.

Helping people change unhealthy behaviour

Changing unhealthy behaviour is successful when the healthy choice becomes the easy choice (Young 2014). A person's health and their health behaviours depend on their physical attributes, together with nonmedical factors. Nonmedical factors can be individual, such as their beliefs, culture, personality, education, income, experiences and circumstances, or social – for example, families, schools, workplaces, communities and the larger political and economic organisation of society (Short & Mollborn 2015). Therefore, for any support with behaviour change to be effective, it must not only address the behaviour, but also the factors surrounding it (Simpson 2015).

Assessing readiness to change

The success, or otherwise, of any intervention to help a person change unhealthy behaviour will partly depend on the person's readiness to change. The Transtheoretical Model of Change (Prochaska & DiClemente 1983) is a tried-and-tested approach to assessing someone's readiness to change. It has six stages:

1. **Precontemplation** – the person does not intend to make any changes soon (usually defined as within the next six months). They are not aware that their behaviour is producing negative consequences. They may underestimate the pros of changing their behaviour and think more about the cons of changing it.

2. **Contemplation** – the person intends to start the healthy behaviour soon. They recognise that their behaviour may be producing negative consequences and they have started to think about the pros and cons of changing the behaviour, giving equal emphasis to each. However, even with this recognition, they may still feel ambivalent about making any changes.

3. **Preparation (Determination)** – the person is ready to make changes (within the next 30 days). They start to take small steps towards the behaviour change and believe this can lead to a healthier life.

4. **Action** – the person has recently changed their behaviour (within the last six months) and they intend to continue with this change. They may show this by modifying their unhealthy behaviour or acquiring new healthy behaviours.

5. **Maintenance** – the person has continued their behaviour change (more than six months) and they intend to maintain this change. They work to prevent themselves relapsing to earlier stages.

6. **Termination** – the person has no desire to return to their unhealthy behaviours and they are sure they will not relapse. This stage is often not considered, as most people tend to stay in the maintenance stage.

Motivating change at each stage of readiness

Empowering and motivating people to generate their own solutions to their problems is the most effective way of sustaining behaviour change (Kelly & Barker 2016). There are several techniques which can encourage people to make positive changes.

One such approach is motivational interviewing (MI), which enables the person to discover and articulate the benefits and costs of change via a gentle process of negotiation. It is a directive, client-centred type of counselling that aims to help people explore and resolve ambivalence about behaviour change. It combines elements of style (warmth and empathy) with technique (reflective listening and the development of discrepancy).

When using this approach, the person does more than 50% of the talking and the healthcare professional focuses on listening. Most of the interventions are summarised, with a few open-ended questions that avoid getting ahead of the person's level of readiness.

There are four central principles in MI:

1. **Express empathy.** The healthcare professional aims to understand the person's issues, struggles, and barriers to change by listening and reflecting. It allows the person to be open as there is a lack of judgement and criticism. An example of a healthcare professional's response might be, 'I can understand why eating lots of cake is tempting in that situation.'

2. **Develop discrepancy.** The healthcare professional aims to get the person to highlight the disparity between what they are doing and what their goals are. This is achieved by asking a series of open questions and encouraging reflection that leads the person to this natural conclusion without any confrontation; for example, if the goal is to be slim and fit, then eating lots of cakes every day may get in the way of that.

3. **Roll with resistance.** Some resistance and reluctance from the person is to be expected. The healthcare professional should not try to force or manipulate the person into acceptance. They should work to understand the person's point of view, avoid the desire to correct what they may see as flawed ways of thinking but offer alternative ways of thinking for them to consider.

4. **Support self-efficacy (a belief in change).** Some people may have tried to change their behaviour previously with limited success, so may be less hopeful about future achievement. The healthcare professional should point to areas of strength and encourage the person to reflect on occasions when they were able to accomplish their goal.

By using this approach, the healthcare professional can identify the person's stage of readiness and then consider the most appropriate therapeutic intervention. For example, if the person is not sure about giving up smoking and is still at the pre-contemplation or contemplation stage, the professional should acknowledge this through empathic listening. The professional should also be curious about the reasons the person wants to stop or not stop smoking. They should not judge and start educating them about cessation methods until the person voices a wish to change. If the healthcare professional advises the person that they are available to help at any time, they are giving them the opportunity to come back if and when they are ready. However, if the person is at the action stage, then it would be appropriate to offer them support to help them change their behaviour.

The healthcare professional's role at each stage of readiness

Here are some examples of interactions between a healthcare professional and a client, at different stages of readiness to change.

1. Pre-contemplation:

Person's response (I'm OK as I am)

'I'm happy being this size'

'My husband likes me cuddly'

'My weight's never bothered me'

Stage of change – pre-contemplation
- No interest in changing
- Very little point in giving health information

Role of the healthcare professional
- Be curious
- Use MI skills, chat and look for discrepancies, listen for any change talk
- If any interest is shown, ask permission to offer advice

For example:
Person: *'I can't exercise because my knees are bad.'*

Response that might cause conflict:
Healthcare professional: *'You could try some non-impact exercise such as swimming or an exercise bike.'*

Response to avoid conflict:
Healthcare professional: *'Oh, I'm sorry to hear that. Are you aware of any exercises that won't affect your knees?'*

Often healthcare professionals will see the solution and the temptation is to offer it instantly. However, if the patient is not ready, they will respond defensively with lots of reasons why they cannot follow the suggestion. This is where conflict can occur.

2. Contemplation:

Person's response (I may want to do something different)
'My rubbish diet does bother me sometimes when I can't get jeans to fit'
'I tried to diet once but all I got was smaller boobs'

Stage of change – pre-contemplation
- Some interest in making a change
- Able to receive information
- Able to discuss barriers

Role of the healthcare professional (decisional balance)
- Be curious and amplify any change talk
- Consider working through the pros and cons of making a change and importantly the benefits and disadvantages of staying exactly as they are

3. Preparation and action:

Person's response (All right I'll give it a go – but how do I start?)
'It has been worrying me a lot lately'
'I think I'll have a go at eating more fruit and veg'

Stage of change – preparation and action
- Planning to change
- Making preparations to have a go

Role of the healthcare professional (enable change)
- Remain curious, refer to leaflets and evidence, tell stories and use narratives
- Help the person to set a goal

4. Maintenance:

Person's response (I've made a few changes – can I stop now?)

'I've lost 3 pounds and can now swim 10 lengths – isn't that enough?'

'It's starting to get quite difficult'

Stage of change – maintenance
- Making changes
- Becoming satisfied
- Maintaining the gains and keeping up with the changes

Role of the healthcare professional (encourage and motivate)
- Listen and reflect on their successes
- Offer more choice regarding ways to achieve the change
- Introduce a new goal to complement their current changes
- Be a mirror to their success
- Encourage positive self-talk

5. Maintenance and relapse prevention:

Person's response (I want to give up)

'I'm really missing cake and booze'

'No one really notices anymore'

Stage of change – maintenance (relapse prevention)
- Losing motivation
- Becoming negative

Role of the healthcare professional (reassure and offer strategies)
- Be curious. 'What are your thoughts about why you feel this way?'
- Revisit the decisional balance
- Review the goal

Supporting people to change their behaviour

The COM-B model describes the elements needed to ensure that any change in behaviour can occur (Michie, van Stralen & West 2011). COM-B is an acronym for Capability, Opportunity, Motivation and Behaviour. According to this model a person must:

- Be physically and psychologically **capable** of performing the necessary actions. This includes having the necessary knowledge and skills.
- Have the physical and social **opportunity** to perform the necessary actions. There may be external factors that make the behaviour impossible.
- Be **motivated** to adopt the new, rather than the old, behaviour, whenever necessary. Motivation is defined as all those brain processes that energise and direct behaviour, not just goals and conscious decision-making.

If one of these components is lacking, the person should be encouraged to choose a different behaviour to work on.

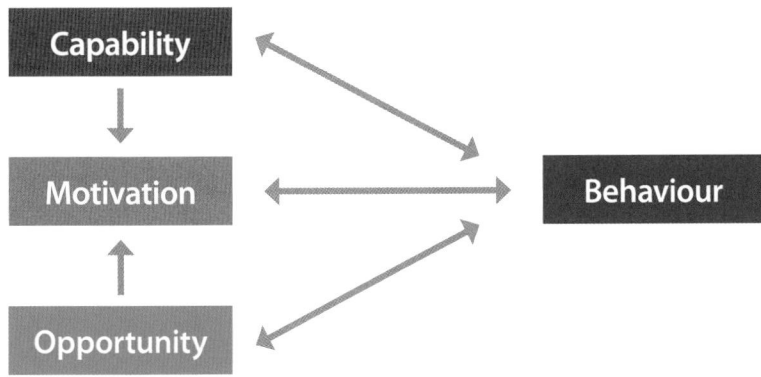

To illustrate, here's an example where all three components are lacking:

Sarah's target is to walk to work three times a week for the next two weeks.

- **Capability** – Sarah has not walked further than the bus stop for years. Her workplace is two miles away. She may not be physically capable of doing this yet. A shorter target distance may be more achievable at this stage.
- **Opportunity** – four out of five days Sarah needs to get to a meeting which is only accessible by car; therefore she will not be able to walk to work on those days.
- **Motivation** – Sarah thinks walking is boring and she does not like getting wet in the rain before going into work. Another form of exercise may be more appealing.

Using a structured approach to support behaviour change

People can be supported to change their unhealthy behaviour using a structured approach (NICE 2019). The methods described here are included in Abraham and Michie's taxonomy of behaviour change techniques (2008):

1. Set the goal
2. Plan the action
3. Record the action
4. Review progress
5. Give positive feedback
6. Support with relapse.

Set the goal

Setting a goal gives something specific for the person to aim for. Achievement is more likely if one goal is set at a time. The goal should be related to a behaviour, e.g. walking. It should also be SMART – that is specific (who, what, where, when, how often, with whom, in what context), measurable (establish criteria), achievable (realistic, attainable, i.e. start small and build up), relevant (the person understands the link between their goal and their desired outcome) and timely (realistic, what works for the person).

The healthcare professional can assist the person to set their own goal. It is helpful to discuss the pros and cons of a possible goal as this may help to overcome initial resistance. Writing down the pros and cons of the goal can be helpful in deciding how achievable it will be.

Required outcome:	
Goal:	
Pros:	**Cons:**

An example:

Outcome: Lose 2 stone

Possible **behaviours** that the patient can choose to lose weight are:

- to increase their physical activity
- or to change their diet.

Goal = the level reached of the chosen behaviour before the next review (e.g. in two weeks will be walking for ten minutes, four times a week, at a gentle pace **OR** in two weeks will have cut down to one packet of crisps a day).

Plan the action

Having a plan helps the person to achieve their goal. Healthcare professionals should encourage the person to link their actions to established routines where possible (e.g. taking medication with breakfast), or to make the new actions become routine. This takes less effort, so success is more likely to be achieved.

There are usually four components to the action plan: where the action is going to take place; when it is going to happen; anyone else involved; and how long the action will take.

Involving others can help people to achieve their goal – for example: going to a stop smoking group, ramblers or slimming club; exercising with a friend; or planning shopping/meals with a partner or flatmate.

An example:

Goal: Mary will walk briskly for 15 minutes three times a week with Angela (her next-door neighbour).

Action plan:
- Set alarm for 7.15 on Sunday, Tuesday and Thursday night and get walking clothes ready.
- Get up at 7.15 (15 minutes earlier than usual) on Monday, Wednesday and Friday.
- Collect Angela at 7.30.
- Walk briskly to the post box (which is about 7 or 8 minutes away) and back again.

Record the action

It is very important that the person records what they have done in their action plan, so they have a realistic picture of their progress. It helps to avoid over- or under-estimation of what they have done. In addition, if they have done well, seeing the evidence of their success will increase their motivation.

Should there be a problem in achieving their goal, this will be identified. The healthcare professional should help the person decide how their chosen action might be measured and encourage them to record this in their plan (e.g. ticks, text, emojis). An appointment to review their progress should be made on a date which matches the target date of their goal.

Action Plan
Target date:
Plan (where, when, who with, for how long):
Record of action:

Review progress

When the person returns to see the healthcare professional, they should be greeted with an open question such as, 'How did you get on last week?' This gives them the opportunity to explain their progress (or lack of progress) as they see it. Questions like 'Did you manage to…?' should be avoided because if they did not reach the goal that was set, it will make them feel that they have failed. The focus should be on what the person has managed to achieve.

Once the person has described their progress in their own words, the healthcare professional can look at their plan. This will help them understand what the person has actually achieved, compared with their perception of what they have achieved.

Response of the healthcare professional if the person has achieved their goal:

- Praise them for their achievement.
- Decide together whether to keep the same goal, to make sure the change that has been achieved is stable, or (if appropriate) set a new goal.

Response of the healthcare professional if the person has partly achieved or not achieved their goal:

- Praise them for any effort made towards achieving their goal (see section on 'giving positive feedback' below).
- Identify anything learnt from the experience that can be used to plan future actions.
- Discuss the other possible actions which may achieve the goal. If other actions cannot be identified, then set a new goal.

Give positive feedback

Giving the person positive feedback will promote their engagement and motivation to continue with their plan. There are two types of feedback that can be given:

1. General positive feedback: 'it's great to see you' or 'well done on last week'
2. Positive feedback on their actions. This can be divided into three forms:
   - Behaviour: 'You've managed an extra walk this week, that's great.'
   - Effort: 'Well done – getting up earlier seems to be helping you get those walks in.'
   - Outcome: 'That's great; you've nearly reached your fitness target!'

Deal with relapse

When the person has relapsed, the healthcare professional should assist them to get back on track and prevent them from feeling that they have failed. The person should be advised that change rarely occurs smoothly, as it is a process rather than an event; and relapse is an opportunity to learn about the situations that are likely to lead to setbacks and what they can do to avoid them. Developing strategies to manage the risky situations will help them to get back on track.

> **Here is an example:**
> Julie's action plan has been to get up earlier on Wednesdays and Fridays and go for a brisk walk. Her friend has started to come round on a Tuesday night and stay late; this has prevented Julie getting up the next day. The healthcare professional asked Julie if she was happy with her friend coming round and staying late. She was, so they discussed the options of changing the Wednesday morning walk to the evening or moving it to a Monday or Tuesday morning. If she had not been happy about the situation, then she would have discussed with Julie how she might approach her friend.

Summary

Healthy behaviour enhances wellbeing, prevents health problems, and can help achieve a positive body image. Healthcare professionals in primary care can help people change unhealthy behaviour by assessing their readiness to change, responding appropriately, and supporting them with a structured approach.

> ## Vignette
> Gordon is 53 years old. He eats lots of takeaways, smokes 10 cigarettes a day and cycles a mile to work each day. His GP has advised him that his blood pressure is high, and he needs to lose weight and stop smoking. Gordon is reluctant to take this advice but wants to be healthy.
>
> How should the healthcare professional approach the consultation?

Reflective questions

- Consider the last time you offered someone support to change unhealthy behaviour
    - o   Were you aware of their stage of readiness to change?
    - o   What might you do differently now in the same situation?
- What could your organisation do to help you support people to change their behaviour?

Answers to 'Is this a behaviour?' on p. 25

a)   Yes

b)   No

c)   Yes

d)   Yes

e)   No

f)   No

g)   Yes

References

Abraham, C. & Michie, S. (2008). A taxonomy of behaviour change techniques used in interventions. *Health Psychology*. **27**, 379–87.

Addictions UK (2020). Addictive behaviour. https://addictionsuk.com/addictive-behaviour/ (Last accessed 26.8.2021).

Alavi, S., Ferdosi, M., Jannatifard, F. *et al.* (2012). Behavioral addiction versus substance addiction: correspondence of psychiatric and psychological views. *International Journal of Preventative Medicine*. **3** (4), 290–294.

Clay, R. (2017). The link between food and mental health. *American Psychological Association*. **48** (8), 26.

Cockerham, W. (2014). Health behavior. *The Wiley Blackwell Encyclopedia of Health, Illness, Behavior and Society*. https://onlinelibrary.wiley.com/doi/epdf/10.1002/9781118410868.wbehibs296 (Last accessed 26.8.2021).

Colten, H. & Altevogt, B. (2006). Eds for the Institute of Medicine (U.S.) Committee on Sleep Medicine and Research, *Sleep Disorders and Sleep Deprivation: An Unmet Public Health Problem*. Washington DC: National Academies Press.

Department of Health (DoH) (2005). Self-care – a real choice: self-care support – a practical option. https://webarchive.nationalarchives.gov.uk/ukgwa/+/dh.gov.uk/en/publicationsandstatistics/publications/publicationspolicyandguidance/dh_4100717 (Last accessed 26.8.2021).

Department of Health (DoH) (2016). UK Chief Medical Officers' Low Risk Drinking Guidelines. https://www.gov.uk/government/uploads/system/uploads/attachment_data/file/545937/UK_CMOs__report.pdf (Last accessed 26.8.2021).

Devore, E., Grodstein, F., Duffy, J. *et al.* (2014). Sleep duration in midlife and later life in relation to cognition. *Journal of the American Geriatrics Society*. **62**, 1073–1081.

Dfarhud, D., Malmir, M. & Khanahmadi, M. (2014). Happiness & health: The biological factors – Systematic review article. *Iranian journal of Public Health*. **43** (11), 1468–1477.

Eliopoulos, C. (2010). *Invitation to Holistic Health*. 2nd edn. Boston: Jones and Bartlett.

Ferreira, M., Sherrington. C., Smith, K. *et al.* (2012). Physical activity improves strength, balance and endurance in adults aged 40–65 years: a systematic review. *Journal of Physiotherapy*. **58** (3), 145–156.

Hirshkowitz, M., Whiton, K., Albert, S.M., *et al.* (2015). National Sleep Foundation's sleep time duration recommendations: methodology and results summary. *Sleep Health*. **1**, 40–43.

Hooker, S. & Masters, K. (2018). Daily meaning salience and physical activity in previously inactive exercise initiates. *Health Psychology*. **37** (4), 344–354.

Jacka, F., O'Neil, A., Opie, R. *et al.* (2017). A randomised controlled trial of dietary improvement for adults with major depression (the 'SMILES' trial). *BMC Medicine*. **15**, 23 https://doi.org/10.1186/s12916-017-0791-y (Last accessed 26.8.2021).

Kelly, M. & Barker, M. (2016), Why is changing health-related behaviour so difficult? *Public Health*. **136**, 109–116. https://doi.org/10.1016/j.puhe.2016.03.030 (Last accessed 26.8.2021).

Kryger, M. (2017). *The Mystery of Sleep*. New Haven: Yale University Press.

Lieberman, H., Carvey, C. & Thompson, L. (2010). Caffeine. In: P. Coates (ed.) *Encyclopedia of Dietary Supplements*. New York: Informa Healthcare USA, Inc.

Marshall, A., Heffernan, T. & Hamilton, C. (2016). The synergistic impact of excessive alcohol drinking and cigarette smoking upon prospective memory. *Frontiers in Psychiatry*. https://www.frontiersin.org/articles/10.3389/fpsyt.2016.00075/full (Last accessed 26.8.2021).

McLellan, T. & Lieberman, H. (2012). Do energy drinks contain active components other than caffeine? *Nutrition Reviews*. **70**, 730–44.

Mehta, N. & Myrskyl, M. (2017). The population health benefits of a healthy lifestyle: Life expectancy increased and onset of disability delayed. *Health Affairs*. 10.1377/hlthaff.2016.1569 (Last accessed 26.8.2021).

Mental Health Foundation (2007). *Feeding minds: the impact of food on mental health*. https://www.mentalhealth.org.uk/sites/default/files/FeedingMinds_exec_summary.pdf (Last accessed 26.8.2021).

Michie, S., van Stralen, M. & West, R. (2011). The behaviour change wheel: A new method for characterising and designing behaviour change interventions. *Implementation Science*. **6**, 42.

National Institute for Health and Care Excellence (NICE) (2019). *Behaviour change: individual approaches.* https://www.nice.org.uk/guidance/ph49/resources/behaviour-change-individual-approaches-pdf-1996366337989 (Last accessed 26.8.2021).

National Institute on Drug Abuse (NIDA) (2020). *Health Consequences of Drug Misuse.* https://www.drugabuse.gov/drug-topics/health-consequences-drug-misuse/introduction (Last accessed 26.8.2021).

NHS (2019). *Exercise.* https://www.nhs.uk/Livewell/fitness/Pages/physical-activity-guidelines-for-adults.aspx (Last accessed 26.8.2021).

NHS (2020). *How smoking affects your body.* https://www.nhs.uk/smokefree/why-quit/smoking-health-problems (Last accessed 26.8.2021).

Orzeł-Gryglewska, J. (2010). Consequences of sleep deprivation. *International Journal of Occupational Medicine and Environmental Health.* **23** (1), 95–114.

Petry, N., Zajac, K. & Ginley, M. (2018). Behavioral addictions as mental disorders: to be or not to be? *Annual Review of Clinical Psychology.* **14**, 399–423.

Planned Parenthood (2020). Six Types of Self-Care. https://secure.everyaction.com/p/Pg5bqblugE6-NGld09RlcQ2 (Last accessed 26.8.2021).

Prochaska, J. & DiClemente, C. (1983). Stages and processes of self-change of smoking: Toward an integrative model of change. *Journal of Consulting and Clinical Psychology.* **51**, 390–395.

Pudikov, I. & Dorokhov, V. (2012). The special physiological importance of the UV-A spectrum for successful phototherapy. *Human Physiology.* **38**, 634–639.

Rehm, J., Baliunas, D. & Borges, G.L.G. *et al.* (2010). The relation between different dimensions of alcohol consumption and burden of disease – an overview. *Addiction.* **105** (5), 817–843.

Short, S. & Mollborn, S. (2015). Social determinants and health behaviors: Conceptual frames and empirical advances. *Current Opinion in Psychology.* **5**, 78–84.

Simpson, V. (2015). *Models and Theories to Support Health Behavior Intervention and Program Planning.* Purdue Extension: Health and Social Sciences. https://extension.purdue.edu/extmedia/hhs/hhs-792-w.pdf (Last accessed 26.8.2021).

Temple, J., Bernard, C., Lipshultz, S. *et al.* (2017). The safety of ingested caffeine: A comprehensive review. *Frontiers in Psychiatry.* **8**, 80. https://doi.org/10.3389/fpsyt.2017.00080 (Last accessed 26.8.2021).

World Health Organization (WHO) (2018). *Physical activity.* http://www.who.int/features/factfiles/physical_activity/en/ (Last accessed 26.8.2021).

Young, S. (2014). Healthy behavior change in practical settings. *The Permanente Journal.* **18** (4), 89–92.

CHAPTER 3

Common mental disorders

Learning outcomes

By the end of this chapter the reader will:

- Know which conditions are defined as common mental disorders
- Be able to screen for depression and anxiety
- Understand how to use tools designed to assess the severity of depression and anxiety
- Know how to assess suicide risk
- Be aware of the treatments available for common mental disorders
- Understand which agencies offer treatment for common mental disorders

Introduction

Common mental disorders (CMD) are described by the National Institute for Health and Care Excellence (NICE 2011), as depression, generalised anxiety disorder (GAD), social anxiety disorder, panic disorder, obsessive compulsive disorder (OCD), and post-traumatic stress disorder (PTSD). The definitions and treatments for each disorder are explained in this chapter, and the responsibilities of healthcare professionals looking after people with CMD in primary care are clarified.

Every seven years in England, the Adult Psychiatric Morbidity Survey (APMS) is carried out. It reports the trends and prevalence of many different mental health problems and treatments (though it does not include PTSD). At the time of writing, the survey was last carried out in 2014 (Stansfeld, Clark, *et al.* 2016). The authors found that nearly half (43.4%) of adults thought they had had a diagnosable mental health condition at some point in their life (35.2% of men and 51.2% of women); but only a fifth of men (19.5%) and a third of women (33.7%) had been given the diagnoses by a healthcare professional. A national survey of wellbeing (Evans, Macrory & Randall 2016) showed that, in 2014, 19.7% of people in the UK over the age of 16 had symptoms of anxiety or depression; this percentage was higher among females (22.5%) than males (16.8%).

Depression

According to a systematic review in 2013 (Vos, Barber, *et al.* 2015), depression was the second leading cause of disability globally, with lower back pain being the first. Depression can negatively affect how a person feels, thinks and behaves. They may feel sad and/or experience a loss of interest in activities they once enjoyed. It can lead to a variety of emotional and physical problems and reduce a person's ability to function both at work and at home. The symptoms and experience of depression vary in every person.

Physical symptoms	Psychological symptoms
• **Change in appetite** • **Change in bowel function** • **Dry mouth** • **Palpitations** • **Indigestion** • **Feeling slowed down** • **Looking unkempt** • **Loss of libido** • **Amenorrhoea (absence of menstruation)** • **Sleep disturbance** • **Headaches, giddiness, sensation of tight band round chest and head, skin-picking, handwringing, general aches and pains**	• **Thinking slow and difficult** • **Poor concentration** • **Preoccupation with morbid thoughts (death/ suicide) and/or physical symptoms** • **Feeling sad, low, or flat** • **Fed up, indecisive** • **Indifference, denial, or lack of awareness of symptoms** • **Loss of interest in life** • **Speech; slow, monotonous, monosyllabic answers; incessant negative talk**

Outcomes are influenced by their personality, resilience, family history, premorbid difficulties (for example, trauma, sexual abuse), relationships and social problems. The National Institute for Health and Care Excellence guidelines for depression (NICE 2009a, reviewed 2013 with update due in 2022) employ the Diagnostic and Statistical Manual (DSM) to define the condition. This is published by the American Psychiatric Association and offers a common language and standard criteria for the classification of mental disorders.

The version described by NICE is the DSM–IV, though it has since updated to DSM-V (American Psychiatric Association 2013). There are nine criteria for diagnosis:

1. Depressed mood most of the day, nearly every day
2. Markedly diminished interest or pleasure in all, or almost all, activities most of the day, nearly every day
3. Significant weight loss when not dieting, or weight gain
4. Insomnia or hypersomnia nearly every day

5. Psychomotor agitation or retardation nearly every day
6. Fatigue or loss of energy nearly every day
7. Feelings of worthlessness or excessive or inappropriate guilt nearly every day
8. Diminished ability to think or concentrate, or indecisiveness, nearly every day
9. Recurrent thoughts of death (not just fear of dying), recurrent suicidal ideation.

Types of depression

There are different types of depression: subthreshold depression, mild depression, moderate depression, major depressive disorder, persistent depressive disorder, seasonal affective disorder and bipolar disorder. Bipolar disorder is classified as a severe mental illness and is covered in Chapter 4.

- Subthreshold depression: fewer than five of the diagnostic criteria
- Mild depression: five or more of the diagnostic criteria and the symptoms result in minor functional impairment
- Moderate depression: five or more of the diagnostic criteria and mild to severe functional impairment
- Major depressive disorder (MDD): also referred to as severe depression, most of the diagnostic criteria, and the symptoms markedly interfere with functioning (this can occur with or without psychotic symptoms)
- Persistent depressive disorder: the person experiences low mood that has lasted for at least two years but may not have reached the intensity of major depression. Often the person can function day to day but feels low or joyless much of the time. They may experience some depressive symptoms, such as appetite and sleep changes, low energy, low self-esteem, or hopelessness.
- Seasonal affective disorder (SAD): this arises when the days get shorter in the autumn and winter. It is thought that the lack of sunlight may affect the hypothalamus and cause it to produce higher levels of melatonin (a hormone associated with sleep) and lower levels of serotonin (a hormone which affects mood, appetite and sleep). The lack of sunlight can also affect the body's circadian rhythm (body clock).

Types of depression that are exclusive to women

Women have a higher rate of general depression than men (Stansfeld *et al.* 2016). Additionally, there are two depression types that are influenced by female reproductive hormones, perinatal depression and premenstrual dysphoric disorder (PMDD). Bipolar disorder is classified as a severe mental illness and is covered in Chapter 4.

- Perinatal depression: this includes major and minor depressive episodes that occur during pregnancy or in the first 12 months after delivery (also known as postpartum depression).
- Premenstrual dysphoric disorder (PMDD): this is a severe form of premenstrual syndrome (PMS). The symptoms usually begin in the late luteal phase of the menstrual cycle (shortly after ovulation) and end once menstruation starts.

Anxiety

It is normal to feel fear in response to a danger or threat. When a person experiences fear, it triggers their 'fight or flight' response. In other words, the body adapts psychologically and physically, enabling the person to either run away or fight to their maximum ability. Anxiety disorders occur when the fight/flight response is triggered inappropriately, so the anxiety is actually a normal reaction to an abnormal stimulus.

This stimulus is often the thought of a threat or something going wrong in the future, but it could also be due to current circumstances. It can lead to the person avoiding the situation that makes them anxious. The person may sometimes think the physical consequences of the fight/flight response (tachycardia, rapid breathing, muscle tension, nausea, trembling) are being caused by a physical illness.

Anxiety disorders can vary in their severity but they all have been associated with significant long-term disability. There may be a lifelong pattern of relapse and remission, and other problems such as depression or substance misuse may also be present.

In 2013, there were 8.2 million known cases of anxiety in the United Kingdom (Fineberg, Haddad, *et al.* 2013). Most anxiety disorders have a relatively early age of onset, with symptoms and syndromes likely to start in childhood or adolescence (NICE 2014). The authors of the NICE quality standard for anxiety (NICE 2014) explain that most anxiety disorders go unrecognised and those that are diagnosed are treated in primary care. Even when anxiety disorders coexist with depression, and the depressive episode is recognised, the underlying and more persistent anxiety disorder is often not detected.

Types of anxiety

Types of anxiety include generalised anxiety disorder (GAD), social anxiety disorder, panic disorder, obsessional compulsive disorder (OCD), and post-traumatic stress disorder (PTSD).

- **Generalised anxiety disorder** is characterised by excessive worry about different events, associated with heightened tension. Symptoms include irritability, restlessness, tiredness, tense muscles, poor concentration and sleeping problems. For the disorder to be diagnosed, symptoms should be present for at least six months and should cause clinically significant distress or impairment in social, occupational or other important areas of functioning (American Psychiatric Association 2013). In 2014, 5.9% of the population in England reported they had this disorder (Stansfeld, Clark, *et al.* 2016).

- **Social anxiety disorder** is a persistent fear of, or anxiety about, one or more social situations that is out of proportion to the actual threat they present. A social situation involves interaction, observation and performance. There are no UK epidemiological surveys that specifically report data on social anxiety disorder in adults, but lifetime prevalence rates of up to 12% have been described in American studies (NICE 2013).

- **Panic disorder** is categorised by recurring unforeseen panic attacks, followed by at least one month of persistent worry about having another panic attack. The symptoms of a panic attack include: heart pounding or racing; dizziness; nausea; chest pain; abdominal pain; difficulty in breathing or a choking sensation; feeling very hot or very cold; sweating, trembling or shaking. There may also be concern about the consequences of a panic attack, or a significant change in behaviour related to the attacks. For a diagnosis, at least two unexpected panic attacks should have occurred that have not been caused by the use of a substance, a general medical condition or another psychological problem (American Psychiatric Association 2013). In 2014, the Adult Psychiatric Morbidity Survey (APMS) found that 0.6% of the population in England had panic disorder (Stansfeld, Clark, *et al.* 2016) and lifetime prevalence rates of 5% have been described in American studies (NICE 2013).

- **Obsessive compulsive disorder (OCD)** is characterised by the presence of obsessions and/or compulsions. An obsession is an unwanted intrusive thought, image or urge that repeatedly enters the person's mind. A compulsion is a repetitive behaviour carried out because the person has an overwhelming feeling that they must do it. The symptoms often cause substantial functional impairment and distress. The APMS reported that 1.3% of England's population had OCD (Stansfeld, Clark, *et al.* 2016).

- **Post-traumatic stress disorder** can develop after a stressful event or situation of an exceptionally threatening or catastrophic nature that is likely to cause pervasive distress in almost anyone (NICE 2018). People might develop the disorder in response to one or more traumatic events such as: serious accidents; physical and sexual assault; abuse, including childhood or domestic abuse; work-related exposure to trauma, including remote exposure; trauma related to serious health problems or childbirth experiences (for example, intensive care admission or neonatal death); war and conflict; and torture. The person may present with a range of symptoms, including re-experiencing, avoidance, hyperarousal (including hypervigilance, anger and irritability); negative alterations in mood and thinking; emotional numbing; dissociation; emotional dysregulation; interpersonal difficulties or problems in relationships; and negative self-perception (including feeling diminished, defeated or worthless).

The responsibility of primary healthcare practitioners

Most people with a mental illness in England are dealt with in primary care (Gask, Kendrick, *et al.* 2018, DoH 2012) yet mental illness is unrecognised in two-thirds of those attending (Mitchell, Vaze & Rao 2009). MIND published a report for Clinical Commissioning Groups in 2016. In it they explain that patients may visit a healthcare professional in primary care and discuss other concerns that are affecting their mental health. It may be a physical health issue or a social matter (such as relationship problems, unemployment or work-related issues, welfare benefits, financial worries or social isolation). They may attend frequently before their underlying mental health needs are addressed.

National guidance advocates that healthcare professionals working in primary care have a responsibility to identify CMD, assess their severity, provide relevant information, and consider any special needs (NICE 2011). They should also offer the correct treatment options for those with mild to moderate problems and make an appropriate referral for those who have a moderate to severe CMD. The National Confidential Inquiry (2018) assert that there should be a mechanism in place to ensure that people who present with major physical health issues are also assessed and monitored for depression and risk of suicide. This is because they are two to three times more likely to have depression than those with good physical health (NICE 2009b, Katon 2011).

Recognising common mental disorders

People with underlying psychological distress may present with a physical health problem such as increased tiredness, bowel problems, difficulties with sleep, headaches or change in appetite. They may also report an increase in smoking, and alcohol or drug consumption. Depression and anxiety are common in people with long-term physical conditions. These individuals may attend to discuss a problem with their long-term condition without realising the cause is psychological. For example, a person with diabetes may attend because their blood glucose readings are raised. This is because they have stopped eating healthily and exercising because they are feeling low.

To ascertain whether someone has depression and/or anxiety, there are screening questions available: two for depression (Whooley, Avins, *et al.* 1997) and two for anxiety (Kroenke, Spitzer & Williams 2001). The person simply answers 'yes' or 'no'; if they answer 'yes' to either question, the healthcare professional should explore whether this is something they want help with and consider further assessment of the mood symptoms they are experiencing. Some primary care practitioners argue that the use of these standardised questions is unnecessary. However, if they are not used, it has been reported that up to seven out of ten cases of depression will go undetected (Arroll, Goodyear-Smith, *et al.* 2005).

As the questions are not written in most people's natural style of conversation, printing the questions on a laminated sheet and asking the person to read them can have a number of benefits: the questions get asked correctly; they have time to think and prepare their response; and they have the option of putting up a barrier between themselves and the healthcare professional while they are thinking. The questions are:

Depression questions:
- 'During the last month have you often been bothered by feeling down, depressed, or hopeless?' **Yes/No**
- 'During the last month have you often been bothered by having little interest or pleasure in doing things?' **Yes/ No**

Anxiety questions:
- 'Do you feel nervous, anxious or on edge?' **Yes/No**
- 'Do you feel unable to stop worrying?' **Yes/ No**

Help question:
- 'Is this something with which you would like help?' **No/Yes, but not today/Yes**

If the person answers 'No' to the first four questions, they are unlikely to have depression or anxiety. The help question improves the specificity of diagnosis; this means if the person answers 'yes' to one of the screening questions and then declines help, this is usually because they do not have underlying depression or anxiety. They should be given the option of coming back to see a healthcare professional if they change their mind.

If the person answers 'Yes' to any of the questions, this should trigger a more detailed assessment, using the Patient Health Questionnaire (PHQ-9) and Generalised Anxiety Disorder Assessment (GAD-7). (See below.)

If a person attends and reports that they are feeling down, depressed or anxious, they can be assessed with the PHQ-9 and GAD-7 (i.e. there is no need to use the screening questions).

When a person screens positively for anxiety or depression, the healthcare professional needs to start by eliminating physical causes and then measure the severity of the depression and/or anxiety.

Eliminating physical causes of depression and/or anxiety

Investigations are not indicated routinely when a person presents with depression but may be necessary to exclude other causes of symptoms. For instance, in someone with predominant fatigue it is useful to carry out a full blood count to exclude anaemia, a thyroid function test to exclude hypothyroidism, and vitamin D to exclude deficiency.

There are some drugs which may cause depressed mood, though this is uncommon. These include:

- Centrally acting antihypertensives (e.g. methyldopa)
- Lipid-soluble beta-blockers (e.g. propranolol)
- Benzodiazepines or other central nervous system depressants
- Opioid analgesics.

Measuring the severity of depression and/or anxiety

Both the PHQ-9 and the GAD-7 tools have been validated for use in primary care.

The PHQ-9 comprises nine questions to score the severity of a person's depression. It is designed to assess their mood over the previous two weeks.

PHQ-9 questions

Over the last two weeks, how often have you been bothered by any of the following problems:

1. **Little interest or pleasure in doing things?**
2. **Feeling down, depressed or hopeless?**
3. **Trouble falling or staying asleep, or sleeping too much?**
4. **Feeling tired or having little energy?**

5. **Poor appetite or overeating?**
6. **Feeling bad about yourself – or that you are a failure or have let yourself or your family down?**
7. **Trouble concentrating on things, such as reading the newspaper or watching television?**
8. **Moving or speaking so slowly that other people could have noticed? Or the opposite – being so fidgety or restless that you have been moving around a lot more than usual?**
9. **Thoughts that you would be better off dead, or of hurting yourself in some way?**

For each of the nine tested criteria, there are four possible answers:

- Not at all   = **0 points**
- Several days   = **1 point**
- More than half the days   = **2 points**
- Nearly every day   = **3 points**

The scores are added up and the depression severity is graded, based on this:

- 0–4   **None**
- 5–9   **mild**
- 10–14   **moderate**
- 15–19   **moderately severe**
- 20–27   **severe**

GAD-7 questions

The GAD-7 contains seven questions to score the severity of a person's anxiety.

Over the last two weeks, how often have you been bothered by any of the following problems:
1. **Feeling nervous, anxious or on edge?**
2. **Not being able to stop or control worrying?**
3. **Worrying too much about different things?**
4. **Having trouble relaxing?**
5. **Being so restless that it is hard to sit still?**
6. **Becoming easily annoyed or irritable?**
7. **Feeling afraid, as if something awful might happen?**

Each question is scored 0–3 in the same way as the PHQ-9. A total score of 1–9 indicates mild anxiety, 10–14 is moderate, and 15–21 is severe. The GAD-7 is only validated to measure the severity of generalised anxiety disorder, i.e. it should not be used to assess social anxiety, panic disorder, OCD or PTSD.

Using both the PHQ-9 and GAD-7 provides only probable diagnoses, so further clinical evaluation is required. The PHQ9 and GAD7 can be used at regular intervals to monitor progress.

Studying the PHQ-9 and GAD-7 questions, for those patients who score 2 or 3 per question, guides the practitioner to choose the most appropriate therapy. The table below provides some examples.

PHQ9 1	**Low-level activity planning (Behavioural Activation – see p. 58)**
PHQ9 2	**Assess suicide risk, consider antidepressant prescription**
PHQ9 3	**Assess sleep hygiene**
PHQ9 4	**Suggest dietary changes/thyroid function test**
PHQ9 5	**Suggest diet advice and keeping a diary**
PHQ9 6	**Consider CBT self-help techniques**
PHQ9 7	**Assign worry time, Behavioural Activation (BA)**
PHQ9 8	**Consider antidepressant prescription**
PHQ9 9	**Assess suicide risk**
GAD7 -1	**Suggest relaxation**
GAD7 -2	**Assign worry time**
GAD7 -3	**Recommend books, e.g. *How to stop worrying and start living* (Carnegie 1993) and computerised CBT**
GAD7 -4	**Suggest relaxation and morning exercise**
GAD7 -5	**Recommend morning exercise**
GAD7- 6	**Keeping a diary for precipitants and challenging critical thinking**
GAD7-7	**Consider CBT self-help techniques**

The Distress Thermometer described in Chapter 1 can be beneficial for people with long-term conditions such as stroke (Gillespie & Cadden 2013) and those with significant language or communication difficulties – for example, people with sensory impairments or a learning disability (NICE 2009b).

Carrying out a biopsychosocial assessment

Mental health and well-being are influenced not only by a person's individual attributes, but also by the social circumstances and environment in which they live. It is therefore important to consider biological, psychological and social factors. The list of questions below is a guide to gaining helpful information:

- What are their current symptoms, including duration and severity?
- Have they had depression before? Is this episode similar to their previous experience?
- Do they have a family history of mental illness? If so, what have they observed and what do they understand?
- What is the quality of their relationships with the people close to them? This may affect their outcome.
- Are they receiving any social support? Are they being given encouragement by family, friends, colleagues, and others? This may be emotional, instrumental (tangible help), informational (advice and suggestions) or appraisal (information that is useful for self-evaluation).
- What are their living conditions? Is this part of the problem?
- Do they have employment and/or financial worries?
- Is there any current or previous alcohol and substance misuse?
- Are they having suicidal thoughts?
- What treatment options are they aware of?
- Have they had any experience of, and response to, treatments? If something has worked in the past, then it may be sensible to use it again.

Suicide

The 2019 Office for National Statistics' bulletin regarding suicide in the UK in 2018 states that there were 6,507 suicides registered in the UK, the first increase since 2013 (ONS 2019). Three-quarters (4,903) of these deaths were men. The highest age-specific suicide rate was for those aged 45 to 49 years (27.1 deaths per 100,000 males and 9.2 deaths per 100,000 females).

The ONS reports that, despite having a low number of deaths overall, rates among the under-25s have generally increased in recent years, particularly in females aged 10 to 24, where the rate has increased significantly since 2012 to its highest level, with 3.3 deaths per 100,000 females. The most common method of suicide in the UK was hanging, which accounted for 59.4% of all suicides among males and 45.0% of all suicides among females.

Suicide is defined by the American Psychiatric Association (2019) as the act of killing yourself, most often because of depression or other mental illness, though this has been disputed (Oquendo & Baca-Garcia 2014). Only half of those who die by suicide have previously been referred to mental health services (National Confidential Inquiry 2013) and one study found that 37% of primary care patients who die by suicide had never received a diagnosis (National Confidential Inquiry 2014).

Suicides can occur impulsively in times of crisis when the person is unable to cope with stress (WHO 2019). Causes of stress may include monetary problems, relationship issues and chronic pain and illness. Other high rates of suicide are prevalent in people who:

- Have experienced conflict (disaster, violence, abuse, loss and a sense of isolation)
- Are discriminated against (refugees and migrants; indigenous peoples; lesbian, gay, bisexual, transgender, intersex [LGBTI] people; and prisoners).
- Have a family history of suicide
- Have made a previous attempt
- Have started antidepressant medication or have had their antidepressant medication changed
- Have a long-term physical condition (or pain)
- Are male
- Are middle-aged
- Abuse alcohol or drugs
- Are under extreme stress
- Self-harm
- Are homeless.

When a person presents with a possible CMD, they should always be asked directly about suicidal thoughts and intent (NICE 2011):

1. **Have you made a suicide attempt in the past?**
   A positive answer should cause you concern.

2. **Do you think that life is not worth living?**
   Many people who are not suicidal think this – it is useful to share with patients that this is a common thought amongst people who are depressed.

3. **Do you think about harming or killing yourself?**
   This is a common thought. A positive response should prompt the remaining questions.

4. **Have you got a plan to kill yourself? How would you do it?**
   If they have no plan there is no need to continue with the questions. If they do, then ask the next question.

5. **Do you aim to carry out this plan?**
   If yes, this person is actively suicidal.

6. **Have you got access to the necessary tools to carry out the plan?**
   Having the tools means the patient has prepared themselves.

7. **What would stop (or is stopping) you from carrying out your plan?**
   Often patients choose not to commit suicide because of commitments to family or friends or faith.

Actions for healthcare professionals

No suicidal thoughts

The healthcare professional should record that an assessment of suicide risk has been made and the person has no suicidal thoughts.

Suicidal thoughts but no plan

The healthcare professional should record that an assessment of suicide risk has been made and the person has suicidal thoughts but no current intent. Any advice and action should also be recorded. The person (and those involved in caring for them) should be advised:

- To immediately seek help (GP, Out of Hours service) if they start to think about making a plan, are concerned, or if their situation deteriorates.
- To contact other sources of help, for example:
    - o Staying safe: https://www.stayingsafe.net/home
    - o The Samaritans: www.samaritans.org Telephone 116 123 (24 hours a day, 7 days a week)
    - o Shout: www.giveusashout.org/ Text Shout to 85258
- To be watchful for changes in mood, negativity and hopelessness, and suicidal intent, particularly during high-risk periods such as initiation of or changes to antidepressant medication or at times of increased stress.

Suicidal thoughts with intent to carry out a plan

The healthcare professional needs to arrange immediate referral to mental health services, following their local procedure. The way this works will vary in different areas of the country and might depend on the person's circumstances. If the suicidal person is accompanied by a friend or family member, they may be asked by the mental health service team to attend one of their locations.

Often the team will come to the practice but there may be a delay. In this situation it is helpful if there is a quiet room in the practice where the person can wait. They should not be left unaccompanied, so having a designated person within the practice (such as an administrator who has been trained to do this) will allow the healthcare practitioner to continue with their clinic.

Treatment for common mental disorders

Treatment for mild to moderate CMD can be offered in the primary care setting. More specialist treatment will require a referral.

Treatments delivered in primary care

CMD treatments that can be provided by healthcare professionals working in primary care include: active monitoring; support to aid physical, psychological and social wellbeing; psychoeducation; and prescribing antidepressants.

Active monitoring

Active monitoring, or watchful waiting, means that the clinician and patient jointly decide not to treat the condition, and to intermittently reassess its status along an agreed follow-up timescale (Hegel, Oxman & Hull 2006). NICE guidance for depression (NICE 2009a) recommends that the follow-up interview should be carried out within two weeks.

Support to aid physical, psychological and social wellbeing

The healthcare professional can help a person with mild to moderate depression to keep well by providing advice, encouragement and support. Some of the approaches listed below are described in Chapter 1.

- **Physical** – sleep hygiene, the benefits of following a regular exercise programme and eating a healthy diet, reducing caffeine and alcohol intake if appropriate, taking medication as prescribed and adequate rest and relaxation.
- **Psychological** – structured problem solving, sharing worries with others, books that can help, listing and estimating, assigning worry time, activity planning, distraction techniques, mindfulness, and self-monitoring diaries.
- **Social** – adult education, meeting up with friends, visiting the library, catching up with relatives, walks in the park and going to the pub for a drink with friends.

Psychoeducation

The aim of psychoeducation is for the person to:
- Learn about their condition and its treatment
- Express how they feel about their condition and its treatment
- Be supported to comply with medication or other treatment
- Recognise their symptoms and crisis situations and know what to do.

Providing a relevant leaflet is a good start – for example:
- Anxiety https://www.nhs.uk/conditions/generalised-anxiety-disorder/
- Depression https://www.nhs.uk/conditions/clinical-depression/

Antidepressant medication

Antidepressant medications are an effective treatment for people with moderate to severe depression. Response to treatment usually occurs within two weeks. Antidepressant medication does not usually work for people with mild depression, so should not normally be prescribed.

In moderate to severe depression, patients will usually need medication to improve their concentration and lift their energy levels before they are able to engage in psychological treatments. People who are newly prescribed antidepressants, or have a change in dose or type, should be reviewed two weeks later to assess the effect. Some antidepressant medication is licensed for anxiety. When it is a first episode of depression, the medication is usually prescribed for at least six months *after* the person reports that they feel better, to prevent relapse. This period may be extended for subsequent episodes.

Selective Serotonin Reuptake Inhibitors (SSRIs) are the most frequently used medicines for the treatment of depression. These include **fluoxetine, citalopram, paroxetine** and **sertraline**. Serotonin (along with noradrenaline and dopamine) is one of the main neurotransmitters in mood disorders; and it has been hypothesised that depression is associated with a lack of serotonin (Cowen & Browning 2015).

Antidepressant drugs exert their effect by boosting serotonin levels in the brain. SSRIs do this by inhibiting the reuptake of serotonin into the neurone, effectively fooling the brain into producing more of the neurotransmitter. It is recommended that healthcare professionals prescribe these first. If there is no response, then a different SSRI should be used before trying another type of antidepressant.

In patients who fail to respond to SSRIs, about half will improve with a different SSRI or class of antidepressant. Alternative classes of antidepressants include:

- Serotonin and Noradrenalin Reuptake Inhibitors (SNRIs)
- Noradrenergic and Specific Serotonergic Antidepressants (NaSSAs)
- Tricyclic antidepressants (TCAs).

Treatment delivered by other agencies

For the person to benefit from treatment delivered by another agency, the healthcare professional will need to make a referral. They need to ensure the referral is appropriate by taking account of patient preference and referring for the least intrusive, most effective intervention first (NICE 2011). If harmful drinking or alcohol dependence is also present, this should be treated first, as it may lead to significant improvement in depressive or anxiety symptoms.

Support or self-help groups

Members of a self-help group share a similar health problem. Their mutual goal is to help each other to manage this problem. Support or self-help groups are often provided by charitable organisations.

Educational and employment support services

Unemployment is linked with poor mental health and being off sick with stress or depression can lead to unemployment (Mental Health Policy Group 2019). A report by Depression Alliance (2016) advocates that local and national health services across the UK must play a greater role in supporting people to find or keep a job, with expanded access to psychological support, an increased number of placement support programmes and further investments in health-led interventions that are proven to work for people with mental health problems. One such initiative, the Mindful Employer, is aimed at increasing awareness of mental health at work and providing support for businesses in recruiting and retaining staff. It is led and supported by employers; more information is available at https://www.mindfulemployer.dpt.nhs.uk/

Individual or group cognitive behavioural therapy

Cognitive (thoughts) behavioural (actions) therapy (CBT) is a psychological intervention where the person works collaboratively with the therapist to learn how their thoughts, beliefs and attitudes affect their feelings and behaviour. They are also taught coping skills to help them deal with different problems.

Individual self-help

Self-help can be facilitated or done alone. It involves the patient using a range of books, manuals and electronic materials based on the principles of CBT.

- **Individual facilitated self-help** – patients are guided by a trained practitioner who introduces the material and reviews their progress and outcomes. The intervention usually consists of six to eight sessions which may be face-to-face and/or conducted by telephone.
- **Non-facilitated self-help** – involves minimal contact with a practitioner (an occasional short telephone call) and includes instructions for the patient to work systematically through the materials over a period of at least six weeks.

Computerised cognitive behavioural therapy

Computerised cognitive behavioural therapy (cCBT) is a form of cognitive behavioural therapy that is delivered through a stand-alone computer-based or web-based programme over a period of nine to twelve weeks. It works best when the patient is facilitated by a trained practitioner who reviews their progress and outcome.

Structured physical activity

Research shows that moderate intensity physical activity interventions, and aerobic activity, if supervised by exercise professionals, can have a positive effect on major depressive disorders (Stanton & Reaburn 2014). Physical activity programmes are defined as structured and group-based (with support from a competent practitioner) and usually comprise three sessions (24–60 minutes' duration) per week for 12 weeks (NICE 2011).

Group-based peer support (self-help) programmes

Peer support can be defined as giving and receiving non-professional, non-clinical assistance from individuals with similar conditions or circumstances (Tracy & Wallace 2016). Some mental health providers commission structured programmes but they are not available everywhere in the country.

Exposure and response prevention

Exposure and response prevention (ERP) is a psychological intervention used for OCD. It aims to help patients overcome their need to engage in obsessive and compulsive behaviours. They are exposed to the feared situation, with the support of a practitioner, and taught ways of coping with their anxiety, distress or fear. The process is repeated until the person no longer feels anxious, distressed or fearful.

Trauma-focused CBT or eye movement desensitisation and reprocessing

Trauma-focused CBT or eye movement desensitisation and reprocessing (EMDR) is a psychological intervention for PTSD. The patient is asked to concentrate on an image connected to the traumatic event and the related negative emotions, sensations and thoughts while watching the therapist's fingers moving from side to side in front of their eyes. After each set of eye movements (about 20 seconds), they are asked to discuss the images and emotions they felt during the eye movements with the therapist. This process is repeated with an emphasis on problematic and persevering memories. When the distress about the image has lessened, they are asked to concentrate on it while having a positive thought relating to it. Treatment should be regular and continuous.

Interpersonal therapy

Interpersonal therapy (IPT) is an intervention that focuses on the patient's interactions. The patient works with the therapist to identify social conflicts, role transitions, grief and loss, and social skills, and their effects on existing symptoms, feelings and problems. They are taught how to cope with or resolve such problems or conflicts. IPT usually consists of 16 to 20 sessions over three to four months.

Behavioural activation

Behavioural activation (BA) is a psychological treatment that aims to reduce symptoms and problematic behaviours through behavioural tasks related to reducing avoidance, activity scheduling, and enhancing positively reinforced behaviours.

Behavioural couples therapy

Behavioural couples therapy aims to help people understand the effects of their interactions with each other, and how their interactions influence the development and continuation of symptoms and problems. The therapy involves working to change the nature of the interactions so that the mental health problems improve.

Counselling

Counselling is a supportive approach which helps patients explore their feelings and problems and make appropriate changes in their lives and relationships.

Short-term psychodynamic psychotherapy

In short-term psychodynamic psychotherapy, the therapist and patient explore conflicts and how these are represented in current situations and relationships, in order to gain understanding. The therapy is non-directive and recipients are not taught specific skills.

Combined interventions

Combined interventions involve the use of more than one type of treatment.

Collaborative care

Collaborative care is a coordinated approach to mental and physical healthcare involving case management, close teamwork between primary and secondary physical health services and specialist mental health services, a range of psychological interventions, and long-term coordination of care and follow-up.

Applied relaxation

Applied relaxation involves the application of muscular relaxation in situations and occasions where the patient is or might be anxious.

Agencies who deliver treatment

Counselling services

Counselling services can be accessed through:

- The workplace – some organisations have telephone or face-to-face provision for their employees
- Charities – counselling may be offered for free, for a donation or for a fixed sum
- Private counsellors – these should be registered with the British Association for Counselling and Psychotherapy (BACP).

Improving Access to Psychological Therapies (IAPT) programme

This service was created to offer patients with mild, moderate, and moderate to severe symptoms of anxiety or depression an easily accessible routine first-line treatment, combined (where appropriate) with medication. The services offered may include CBT, IPT, self-help, psychodynamic psychotherapy, EMDR, BA and relaxation. The local IAPT service can be located via the NHS website https://www.nhs.uk/service-search/other-services/Psychological%20therapy%20(NHS%20IAPT)/LocationSearch/396

Third sector organisations

Third sector organisations are nongovernmental organisations (also known as the voluntary sector, community sector or 'not-for-profit' sector). They are called 'third sector', to distinguish them from the public sector (providing basic government services) and the private sector (run by individual groups for profit). Many of these voluntary organisations provide invaluable services for people with mental health problems.

Secondary care mental health services

Secondary care refers to services provided by health professionals who generally do not have the first contact with a person. A GP referral is required to access help from these members of the mental health team. Their roles and functions are described below.

Psychiatrists

A psychiatrist is a medical doctor with specialist training in diagnosing and treating mental illnesses and emotional problems. Each team has a consultant who has completed their professional training. If the patient in contact with specialist mental health services needs to take medication, psychiatrists are usually responsible for prescribing this (although in some services, nurse prescribers take this responsibility too). There may also be an associate specialist, who will have trained in psychiatry but who has not become a consultant.

Community mental health nurses

Community mental health nurses (CMHNs) work outside hospitals and visit people in their own homes, out-patient departments, or GP surgeries. They can help people talk through problems and give practical advice and support. They can also give medicines and review their effects. Nurse therapists have had extra training in particular problems and treatments, such as eating disorders or behaviour therapy.

Social workers

Social workers help people to talk through their problems, give them practical advice and emotional support and provide some psychological treatments. They give expert practical help with money, housing problems and other entitlements.

Occupational therapists

Occupational therapists (OTs) help people get back to undertaking the tasks of everyday life – for example, by doing practical things or talking to other people in groups.

Clinical psychologists

Clinical psychologists will usually meet regularly with a person for a number of sessions to talk through how they are feeling, thinking and behaving. They may use cognitive behavioural therapy, psychodynamic or behavioural psychotherapies. They also advise other members of the mental health team.

Team managers

The team manager will usually be a senior nurse or social worker.

Approved mental health professionals

The approved mental health professional (AMHP) will usually be a social worker but can be any member of the community mental health team. They have had further training in applying the Mental Health Act and have a central role in assessing and determining if there are grounds to compulsorily admit and detain someone in hospital under the Act.

Care coordinators

A person receiving help from secondary care would usually be allocated a care coordinator who is often a social worker or a nurse.

Specialist community-based teams

Some areas in the United Kingdom may have specialist teams, these include:

- Home treatment
- Crisis intervention
- Early onset psychosis
- First episode psychosis
- Assessment and brief treatment (ABT)
- Continuing care
- Recovery
- Assertive outreach
- Forensic
- Child and adolescent mental health.

Healthcare professionals should have an up-to-date record of the contact details of the services they may refer to.

Local service	Contact details
Counselling services	
IAPT service	
Third sector agencies	
Secondary care services	
Other (e.g. social services, debt counselling)	

Summary

Healthcare professionals in primary care have a responsibility to recognise CMD, provide information about the treatment options, and make appropriate referrals. They can also help people with CMD to improve their physical, psychological and social wellbeing.

Vignette

Janet is 43 years old and has attended the practice for her annual diabetes review. She has put on 10 kilograms since last year and her blood glucose is raised. Janet normally exercises regularly and eats a healthy diet. She reports that she is comfort eating and cannot be bothered to exercise or prepare food. She is avoiding eye contact and her reactions appear slow.

How should the healthcare professional approach the consultation?

Review progress

- Think about the last time you were feeling low for a couple of days. How did this affect you physically and mentally?
- What local third sector agencies are available for people with CMD and how can they be accessed?
- What psychological therapies are offered by your local IAPT service? How long do people usually have to wait before they gain access to this treatment and what support do they receive while they are waiting?

References

American Psychiatric Association (APA) (2013). *The Diagnostic and Statistical Manual of Mental Disorders*. 5th edn. Arlington VA: APA.

American Psychiatric Association (APA) (2019). *Suicide*. https://www.apa.org/topics/suicide/ (Last accessed 28.8.2021).

Arroll, B., Goodyear-Smith, F., Kerse, N., Fishman, T. & Gunn, J. (2005). Effect of the addition of a 'help' question to two screening questions on specificity for diagnosis of depression in general practice: diagnostic validity study. *British Medical Journal*. **331** (7521), 884.

Carnegie, D. (1993). *How to Stop Worrying and Start Living*. 3rd edn. London: Cedar.

Cowen, P. J. & Browning, M. (2015). What has serotonin to do with depression? *World Psychiatry: Official Journal of the World Psychiatric Association (WPA)*. **14** (2), 158–160.

Department of Health (DoH) (2012). *Preventing suicide in England: a cross-government outcomes strategy to save lives*. London: DoH.

Depression Alliance (2016). Improving employment outcomes for people with depression. https://aware-ni.org/images/Work_in_Progress_UK_Report.pdf (Last accessed 7.9.2021).

Evans, J., Macrory, I. & Randall, C. (2016). *Measuring national well-being: Life in the UK, 2016*. ONS. https://www.ons.gov.uk/peoplepopulationandcommunity/wellbeing/articles/measuringnationalwellbeing/2016#how-good-is-our-health (Last accessed 28.8.2021).

Fineberg, N., Haddad, P., Carpenter, L., *et al*. (2013). The size, burden and cost of disorders of the brain in the UK. *Journal of Psychopharmacology*. **27**(9), 761–770.

Gask, L., Kendrick, T., *et al*. (2018). *Primary Care Mental Health*. 2nd ed. London: Royal College of Psychiatrists.

Gillespie, D. & Cadden, A. (2013), The Distress Management System for Stroke (DMSS): an approach for screening and initial intervention for post-stroke psychological distress. *Journal of Nursing Education and Practice*. **3** (10), 150–158.

Hardy, S. (2015). Mindfulness: Enhancing physical and mental health wellbeing. *Practice Nursing*. **26** (9), 450–453.

Hegel, M., Oxman, T., Hull, J. *et al*. (2006). Watchful waiting for minor depression in primary care: remission rates and predictors of improvement. *Gen Hosp Psychiatry*. **28**, 205–12.

Katon, W. (2011). Epidemiology and treatment of depression in patients with chronic medical illness. *Dialogues in Clinical Neuroscience*. **13**, 7–23.

Kroenke, K., Spitzer, R. & Williams, J. (2001). The PHQ-9: validity of a brief depression severity measure. *Journal of General Internal Medicine*. **16** (9), 606–613.

McManus, S., Meltzer, H. & Brugha, T. *et al*. (2009). *Adult psychiatric morbidity in England, 2007: results of a household survey*. Leeds: NHS Information Centre for Health and Social Care.

Mental Health Policy Group (2019). *Towards Equality for Mental Health: Developing a Cross-Government Approach*. https://www.nhsconfed.org/sites/default/files/media/Towards%20Equality%20for%20Mental%20Health_2.pdf (Last accessed 7.9.2021).

MIND (2016). Mental Health in Primary Care: A briefing for Clinical Commissioning Groups. https://www.mind.org.uk/media-a/4409/13296_primary-care-policy_web_op.pdf

Mitchell, A., Vaze, A. & Rao, S. (2009). Clinical diagnosis of depression in primary care: a meta-analysis. *Lancet*. **374**, 609–619.

National Confidential Inquiry (2013). *National Confidential Inquiry into Suicide and Homicide by People with Mental Illness. Annual Report, England, Northern Ireland, Scotland and Wales*. Manchester: University of Manchester.

National Confidential Inquiry (2014). *National Confidential Inquiry into suicide and homicide by people with mental illness: suicide in primary care in England: 2002–2011*. Manchester: University of Manchester.

National Confidential Inquiry (2018). *Safer services: a toolkit for specialist mental health services and primary care*. Available at: https://www.rcpsych.ac.uk/docs/default-source/improving-care/nccmh/suicide-prevention/safer-services_a-toolkit-for-specialist-mental-health-services_updated-nov-2018.pdf?sfvrsn=f6620787_2 (Last accessed 28.8.2021).

National Institute for Health and Clinical Excellence (NICE) (2009a). *Depression in adults: recognition and management*. https://www.nice.org.uk/guidance/cg90 (Last accessed 28.8.2021).

National Institute for Health and Care Excellence (NICE) (2009b). *Depression in adults with a chronic physical health problem: recognition and management.* http://www.nice.org.uk/guidance/CG91 (Last accessed 28.8.2021).

National Institute for Health and Care Excellence (NICE) (2011). *Common mental health problems: Identification and pathways to care.* https://www.nice.org.uk/guidance/cg123 (Last accessed 28.8.2021).

National Institute for Health and Care Excellence (NICE) (2013). *Social anxiety disorder. The NICE guideline on recognition, assessment and treatment.* https://www.nice.org.uk/guidance/cg159/evidence/full-guideline-189895069 (Last accessed 28.8.2021).

National Institute for Health and Care Excellence (NICE) (2014). *Anxiety disorders: Quality standard (QS53).* https://www.nice.org.uk/guidance/qs53 (Last accessed 28.8.2021).

National Institute for Health and Care Excellence (NICE) (2018). *Post-traumatic stress disorder.* https://www.nice.org.uk/guidance/ng116/chapter/Recommendations (Last accessed 28.8.2021).

Office for National Statistics (ONS) (2019). *Suicides in the UK: 2018 registrations.* https://www.ons.gov.uk/peoplepopulationandcommunity/birthsdeathsandmarriages/deaths/bulletins/suicidesintheunitedkingdom/2018registrations (Last accessed 28.8.2021).

Oquendo, M. & Baca-Garcia, E. (2014). Suicidal behavior disorder as a diagnostic entity in the DSM-5 classification system: advantages outweigh limitations. *World Psychiatry.* **13** (2), 128–130.

Smiley, E. (2005). Epidemiology of mental health problems in adults with learning disability: an update. *Advances in Psychiatric Treatment.* **11**, 214–222.

Stansfeld, S., Clark, C., Bebbington, P. *et al.* (2016). Chapter 2: Common mental disorders. In: S. McManus, P. Bebbington, R. Jenkins & T. Brugha (eds.) *Mental Health and Wellbeing in England: Adult Psychiatric Morbidity Survey 2014.* Leeds: NHS Digital.

Stanton, R. & Reaburn, P. (2014). Exercise and the treatment of depression: a review of the exercise program variables. *Journal of Science and Medicine in Sport.* **17** (2), 177–182.

Tracy, K. & Wallace, S. (2016). Benefits of peer support groups in the treatment of addiction. *Substance Abuse and Rehabilitation.* **7**, 143–154.

Vos, T., Barber, R., Bell, B. *et al.* (2015). Global, regional, and national incidence, prevalence, and years lived with disability for 301 acute and chronic diseases and injuries in 188 countries, 1990–2013. *Lancet.* **386** (9995), 743–800.

Whooley, M., Avins, A., Miranda, J. & Browner, W. (1997). Case-finding instruments for depression. Two questions are as good as many. *Journal of General Internal Medicine.* **12** (7), 439–445.

Wolf, J. (2018). *The Patient Experience Consumer Study 2018.* Nashville: The Beryl Institute.

World Health Organization (WHO) (2019). *Suicide.* https://www.who.int/news-room/fact-sheets/detail/suicide (Last accessed 28.8.2021).

CHAPTER 4

Severe mental illness

Learning outcomes

By the end of this chapter the reader will:

- Understand how a person is affected by severe mental illness
- Know how to work with a person with severe mental illness
- Recognise relapse in mental health
- Be aware of the physical health issues in severe mental illness
- Consider how to make appointments accessible
- Be able to monitor physical health in severe mental illness
- Appreciate the importance of supporting behaviour change

Introduction

Severe mental illness (SMI) refers to conditions where psychosis is present. Included on the primary care SMI register should be all patients with psychosis, schizophrenia, or bipolar disorder. Around 6% of the population report experiencing at least one indication of psychosis (McManus, Bebbington, *et al.* 2016). Schizophrenia affects less than 1% of people during their lifetime, and around 2% of the population have experienced symptoms of bipolar disorder (MHFA England 2019). Psychosis and schizophrenia typically first occur in young people between the ages of 15 and 30 (Drake, Addington, *et al.* 2016) while bipolar disorder often starts between adolescence and mid-thirties (Dagani, Baldessarini, *et al.* 2019).

How a person is affected by severe mental illness

The way a person is affected by their mental illness influences how they behave and communicate, their ability to organise themselves and their understanding of any information and advice offered. This needs to be taken in to account when planning to see people with SMI.

Psychosis

Psychosis is not a condition but a symptom of mental illness. As the senses are altered, the affected person may not be able to distinguish between reality and their symptoms, and they may perceive or interpret things differently from those around them.

The two main features of psychosis are hallucinations and delusions. When a person experiences a hallucination, they may see, hear, smell, taste or feel something that does not exist. Auditory hallucinations are the most common type; the person might hear someone speaking to them or telling them to do certain things. The voice may be angry, neutral or warm.

A delusion is a belief that is maintained despite being contradicted by reality. Often, there is an element of paranoia. A person experiencing a persecutory delusion may believe they are being spied on, or forced to do something against their will, or that someone is planning to hurt them. Those with a grandiose delusion may believe that they have some sort of power or authority. As people who have psychotic episodes are often unaware that their hallucinations or delusions are not real, they may feel frightened or distressed.

Schizophrenia

Schizophrenia is a psychotic disorder in which the person has positive, negative and cognitive symptoms. The positive symptoms include hallucinations, delusions and disordered thoughts (thoughts and conversation appear illogical and lacking in sequence). The negative symptoms are an absence of behaviour that the person may have had previously. For instance, they may appear emotionally inexpressive and unresponsive, have poor speech, lack a desire for company, be unable to show or feel pleasure, and have a lack of will, spontaneity and initiative. Cognitive symptoms are frequently experienced and may include problems with concentration and task planning.

Bipolar disorder

Bipolar disorder is characterised by episodes of elated mood, known as mania, and episodes of depression. During a manic phase, the person may feel euphoric and self-important, be full of energy and have new ideas, and plans. They often talk quickly, are easily distracted, irritated or agitated, and do not sleep or eat. They may participate in pleasurable behaviour with upsetting consequences, such as spending large amounts of money or engaging in risky sexual encounters.

During the depression phase, the symptoms can include feeling sad and hopeless, empty or worthless, and guilty or despairing. The person may lack energy, have difficulty concentrating and remembering things, lose interest and enjoyment in everyday activities and experience self-doubt. Difficulties with sleeping and waking up early, and suicidal thoughts may also be present. Symptoms of psychosis can be experienced during the mania or depression phase.

Working with a person with severe mental illness

People with severe mental illness should be treated by healthcare professionals in the same way as any other person, in terms of responding to their individual needs. However, some people with SMI can become overwhelmed by their environment, so communicating with them effectively will put them at ease and make good use of the consultation time.

Following some general guidelines can help people feel more comfortable:

- Don't crowd their personal space.
- Show acceptance by saying, for example, 'It's really good to see you.'
- Convey interest, concern and alertness through body posture and facial expression.
- Listen actively – use eye contact, nodding and open gestures. Paraphrase what is being said to ensure mutual understanding.

Most of the time, people with SMI will respond to a healthcare professional in the same way as anyone else, but sometimes the healthcare professional's queries and conversation may be met with silence or monosyllabic answers. Even though they are interested in what is being discussed, the person's facial expression and tone might not convey this. At times, the person with SMI may react in a way that is hard to deal with. Below are some common reactions and how the healthcare professional could respond.

Reaction of person with SMI	How the healthcare professional could respond
Uncommunicative and appearing uninterested.	Continue the conversation until the person shows disapproval.
Displaying odd ways of speaking or behaving.	Attention should not be drawn to this, and the person should not be asked why they are behaving in such a manner. The conversation should be continued normally.
Presenting with inappropriate emotions.	If this causes discomfort or embarrassment to the healthcare professional, or the person does not appear to be managing, the conversation can be postponed to a later time.
Being suspicious of the healthcare professional's intentions and getting angry.	The subject upsetting the person should be avoided. The person should be reassured that the healthcare professional cares for them and would like to continue the conversation when the person is ready to do so.
Displaying unusual behaviour which is affecting the healthcare professional's ability to work with them.	Look at the person. Say exactly what the person is doing that is making the consultation difficult. For example, 'It makes me feel a bit nervous when you keep getting up and walking around the room.'

Recognising relapse in mental health

As with long-term physical conditions, people with SMI may have periods when they relapse. Some reasons for this may include:

- Having a poor understanding of their own condition
- Being unable to recognise the symptoms that indicate when they are becoming unwell
- Not taking their medication as prescribed
- Misusing alcohol or drugs
- Having a poor sleep pattern
- Being stressed
- Not having supportive family and/or friends
- Experiencing stigma
- Having poor physical health.

What to look out for

People with SMI should have a plan in their records which identifies their individual signs and symptoms of a possible relapse and describes the action to be taken by themselves, their family and healthcare professionals. Each person will display different warning signs, but the most common ones to look out for are:

- Mood changes
- Loss of humour
- Irritability and/or agitation
- Losing concentration
- Not joining in
- Talking or acting inappropriately
- Describing strange plans or ideas
- Neglect of personal care
- Dressing in unusual clothes or unusual combinations of clothes (different from their usual attire)
- Appearing more sleepy or lively than usual
- Noticeable weight loss or gain
- Appearing suspicious or hostile
- Intolerant of noise
- Appearing distracted, looking around (maybe be hearing voices or seeing things).

If a person with SMI appears to be relapsing, they should be encouraged to access help. If they are very unwell, they may not recognise that they need help so the healthcare professional should contact their community mental health worker or GP as appropriate.

Physical health in severe mental illness

Both an international study (Firth, Siddiqi, *et al.* 2019) and one carried out in the United Kingdom (Hayes, Marston, *et al.* 2017) found a mortality gap between people with SMI and the general population of up to 25 years. Research has shown that 75% of this excess mortality is likely to be caused by physical illness such as respiratory disease, diabetes and cardiovascular disease (Barber & Thornicroft 2018, Liu, Daumit, *et al.* 2017). Premature mortality in this group can be amplified by economic disadvantage, unhelpful health behaviours (smoking, poor diet, lack of exercise, alcohol misuse), and difficulties accessing and adhering to medical treatments (Olfson, Gerhard, *et al.* 2015).

The antipsychotic medication used to treat SMI is also linked with premature mortality, as it contributes to the development of cardiovascular disease, diabetes and obesity (Torniainen, Mittendorfer-Rutz, *et al.* 2015, Mitchell, Vancampfort, *et al.* 2013). In addition, people with SMI are often not given adequate treatment for major medical conditions which may increase this risk (Woodhead, Ashworth, *et al.* 2016). People with SMI who neglect themselves have the highest mortality rates (Wu, Chang, *et al.* 2012). Yet, when they are at low risk of self-harm or violence, they are often discharged to primary care where enhancing self-care is unlikely to be considered (Hotopf & McCracken 2014).

The mortality gap between people with SMI and the general population has not improved despite increased awareness of the significance of physical comorbidity (Mitchell, Vancampfort, *et al.* 2013). To increase the life expectancy of people with mental health problems, inadequate social relationships, poor housing, unemployment and despondency all need to be addressed, as these factors have a major impact on physical health; but often the focus is on lifestyle factors alone (Marmot 2010).

In addition to conditions causing early mortality, there is a high prevalence of other physical disorders, such as sexually transmitted infections, erectile dysfunction, obstetric complications, osteoporosis, and dental problems in people with SMI (De Hert, Correll, *et al.* 2011). People with SMI are more likely to have metastases at diagnosis and die prematurely from cancer than the general population and less likely to receive specialised interventions for cancer (Bushe, Taylor & Haukka 2010, Kisely, Crowe & Lawrence 2013). The symptoms of physical conditions are often not considered or are viewed by healthcare professionals as part of the person's mental illness (Nash 2013).

Making appointments accessible

People with SMI need to be valued by healthcare professionals as much as those with physical health problems in order to close inequalities in mortality, morbidity and delivery of care (Mitchell, Hardy & Shiers 2017). To achieve this, the government has placed a legal responsibility on health services to make practical modifications to ensure that people with SMI are not disadvantaged, compared with the general population, in accessing healthcare (Equality Act 2010). One way of achieving equality in primary care is to make appointments more accessible for this group by adapting the way they are invited for appointments and the way the appointment is set up.

Inviting people with SMI for a health check

People can be invited by letter and/or telephone or via a prompt from a third party.

Letter invitations

The capacity of people with SMI to remember the appointment or keep to time may be affected by the symptoms of their mental illness, or they may feel too anxious to attend. They may choose not to go to their health check as they are not always made aware of their increased risk of cardiovascular disease and other physical conditions (Hardy, Deane & Gray 2013). This is no different to people without a mental illness who are often not motivated to attend for a check-up when they are uninformed of their health risks (Burgess, Wright, *et al.* 2015).

Several studies in England have shown poor uptake for health checks in the general population, following a standard invitation letter (McDermott, Wright, *et al.* 2016, Norman & Conner 1993). A letter offering a person an appointment with a specific date and time for a health check significantly increases attendance, compared to letters containing an open invitation (Norman & Conner 1993, Camilloni, Ferroni, *et al.* 2013).

The situation appears to be no different for the SMI population; an audit of one primary care practice found that people with SMI had a 70% attendance rate for their physical health check when they were invited by letter giving a date, time, place and name of practitioner (Hardy & Gray 2012). The authors agreed that providing a predetermined date and time removed a complicated step in the process for the person with SMI. Perron, Dao, *et al.* (2010) report increased attendance in the general population following a prompt letter being sent a few days before the appointment. The letter consisted of a short paragraph, which takes about 30 seconds to read, explains the programme of care, and provides gentle encouragement.

Telephone invitations

Randomised controlled trials in England on the subject of NHS health checks showed that more people attended an appointment when invited by telephone, compared to those who received a letter (Gidlow, Ellis, *et al.* 2019), and endorsed text message reminders had a big influence on participation (Sallis, Sherlock, *et al.* 2019).

However, a systematic review of telephone prompting (McClean, Booth, *et al.* 2016) only found one study specific to people with SMI (Reda & Makhoul 2001); they observed no clear difference in attendance between those prompted by telephone one or two days before their appointment and those given appointments via a standard management system. This study took place at a time when people with SMI would have been less likely to have access to a working phone. It is now more common for people to own a mobile phone, with 94% of people in advanced economies being in possession of one (Pew Research Center 2019).

Prompts from a third party

The community mental health team (CMHT) can be advised of the appointment if the person with SMI is in contact with them. They may be able to encourage the patient to come, and in some circumstances one of their team members might attend the appointment too. National guidance for schizophrenia and bipolar disorder asserts that it is the responsibility of the mental health team to ensure that people under their care receive physical healthcare from primary care (NICE 2014a).

Setting up appointments

Practice nurses have made some practical changes to make it easier for people with SMI to attend for their health check, though there is currently no evidence available to show the effects of the measures they have taken. These changes include the time and duration of appointment and having a quiet area for waiting.

- **Time of appointment:** People with SMI may find it difficult to get up due to their symptoms and medication side effects, so avoiding early morning appointments is helpful.
- **Duration of appointment:** People with SMI may struggle with prolonged appointments which offer too much information, although there is a risk of them not coming back if all actions are not completed. It may be helpful to ensure the information given is concise, explain the benefits of returning, and book any follow-up appointments during the consultation.
- **Quiet waiting area:** People with SMI may become agitated if they have to wait, and their anxiety may increase if the waiting room is full of people and is very noisy. This can be avoided by having a separate quiet waiting area, or by organising appointments at a time of day which is not busy.

Monitoring physical health in severe mental illness

According to National Institute for Health and Care Excellence (NICE) guidance for psychosis and schizophrenia (NICE 2014a, checked March 2019) and bipolar disorder (2014b, checked October 2017 and amended February 2020), GPs and other primary healthcare professionals in England should monitor the physical health of people with SMI. The physical health check should be carried out annually when responsibility for monitoring is transferred from secondary care.

Nurses and other primary healthcare professionals will be familiar with most of the recommended features of the annual health check, as they are not dissimilar to those advised for other long-term conditions. Hardy (2013) recommends that a health check in primary care should consist of measurements, blood tests, screening, lifestyle, medication review and a care plan. A manual describing each element in detail is available from a website designed for primary healthcare professionals carrying out these health checks (http://physicalsmi.webeden.co.uk/). This website also has other useful information and tools.

Measurements

Body mass index and/or waist circumference, blood pressure and pulse should be measured. Electrocardiography (ECG) should be performed on all patients with an increased pulse above 100 beats per minute and on those prescribed high doses of antipsychotic medication.

Blood tests

Liver function, lipids, glucose and/or HbA1c should be tested. It is also worth considering whether to test prolactin, urea, electrolytes and calcium, thyroid function, full blood count, B12 and folate, and plasma levels (as appropriate, such as lithium).

Screening

Discuss dental hygiene and dental visits and recommend regular visits to the optician. It is worth examining the person's feet for neglect. Ask if there are problems with urination and enquire about bowel habits. Provide information and instruction about self-examination (testicles, breasts). In women, check cervical cytology has been carried out and ask about their menstrual cycle. Offer advice as appropriate.

Lifestyle

As with other physical conditions, advice and support should be offered as appropriate regarding sleep, smoking, exercise, alcohol, diet and fluids, caffeine and drug use and sex. There are some special considerations to consider in people with SMI when supporting them to reduce or stop smoking (Campion, Francis, *et al.* 2005).

- Smoking increases the metabolism of some medications, including antidepressants, antipsychotics, benzodiazepines and opiates. (This means that the medication leaves the person's system quicker and is less effective.) The doses of these medications may therefore need to be reduced when smoking is reduced to prevent toxicity, with further dose reductions as required with continued cessation.
- Monitor for smoking resumption as original doses of medication need to be reinstated if smoking is restarted.
- Monitor the mental state of people following reduction/cessation (see p. 120). For those taking bupropion and varenicline, there should be a clearly negotiated plan of support that outlines actions to be taken in the event of a change in psychiatric symptoms, especially in the first two to three weeks.

Medication review

All prescribed medication should be reviewed in the usual manner. Most people with schizophrenia will be treated with antipsychotic medication which can be divided into two types: typical (older) and atypical (newer):

- Typical antipsychotics include chlorpromazine, flupentixol, haloperidol, perphenazine, pimozide, prochlorperazine, promazine, sulpiride, trifluperazine, zuclopenthixol

- Atypical antipsychotics include amisulpride (brand name Solian), aripiprazole (Abilify), clozapine (Clozaril, Denzapine, Zaponex), olanzapine (Zypadhera, Zyprexa), paliperidone (Invega, Xeplion), quetiapine (Seroquel, Seroquel XL), risperidone (Risperdal, Risperdal Consta).

Treatment of bipolar disorder depends on how the condition affects the individual patient. Different medication is used in each phase.

Acute manic phase:

- Antipsychotics (olanzapine, quetiapine, risperidone and aripiprazole)
- Valproate, Lithium or Carbamazepine
- PRN benzodiazepines

Depressive phase:

- Selective Serotonin Reuptake Inhibitors (SSRIs), e.g. citalopram, fluoxetine
- Antipsychotics
- Valproate, Lithium or Lamotrigine

Promoting concordance

As with any long-term condition requiring medication, patients are often reluctant to continue taking their treatment for various reasons. It's helpful to follow this list of points when undertaking a medication review:

1. Provide information regarding their condition.
2. Advise on how important it is to take their medication as prescribed and not to miss doses.
3. Ask patient about the type, severity and duration of side-effects. A tool can be used, such as the Glasgow Antipsychotic Side-effect Scale, often referred to as GASS (Waddell & Taylor 2008). Using this can help identify what specific problems the person is suffering from.
4. Explore resistance to therapy.
5. Anticipate that the person may be misinformed about the illness or the treatment.
6. Educate them to continue taking medications when they are feeling better and explain why maintenance treatment is important.
7. Refer the person to their GP or original prescriber as appropriate if they have side effects or are unhappy about their medication.

Long-acting antipsychotic injections

Antipsychotics can be administered either orally or as an injection. There are several reasons why injections may be prescribed instead of tablets:

- It is easier for some patients to have one injection fortnightly or monthly, rather than remembering to take tablets every day

- The exact amount of medication that will be taken, according to the prescription
- When a patient has malabsorption, an injection may be more effective
- There is a steady therapeutic medication level from regular injections
- There is protection from relapse beyond the time of the last injection.

Monitoring lithium

To avoid harm to the recipient, the dosage of lithium needs to be adjusted, based on regular blood tests (usually every three months). The blood level of lithium is dependent on renal function; and lithium has the potential to interfere with both renal and thyroid functions. Additionally, clinically significant alterations in lithium blood levels occur with commonly prescribed and over-the-counter medicines. People with SMI who are taking lithium should be made aware of the known side effects and symptoms of toxicity.

Side effects	Toxic (Medical emergency)
<ul><li>Gastric disturbance</li><li>Mild hand tremor</li><li>Ankle swelling</li><li>Thirst, polyuria</li><li>Metallic taste</li><li>Hypothyroidism</li><li>Disturbed renal function</li></ul>	<ul><li>Severe tremor</li><li>Stomach-ache with nausea and diarrhoea</li><li>Muscle weakness</li><li>Unsteadiness</li><li>Muscle twitching</li><li>Slurring of speech</li><li>Blurred vision</li><li>Confusion</li><li>Sleepiness</li></ul>

Blood tests for urea and electrolytes, including calcium, estimated glomerular filtration rate (eGFR) and thyroid function, should be taken every six months, and more often if there is evidence of impaired renal or thyroid function, raised calcium levels or an increase in mood symptoms that might be related to impaired thyroid function. The person should be monitored at every appointment for symptoms of neurotoxicity, including paraesthesia, ataxia, tremor and cognitive impairment, which can occur at therapeutic levels of lithium.

Care plan

As most patients who have a mental illness are seen only in a primary care setting, it is important that the primary care team takes responsibility for discussing and documenting a plan of care to prevent relapse (NICE 2014a). This should include:

- Current health status
- Social care needs, including how needs are to be met
- Social support – for example, help from friends or family or voluntary organisations

- Summary of services received from secondary care
- Occupational status
- 'Early warning signs' that may indicate a possible relapse
- The patient's preferred course of action (discussed when well) in the event of a clinical relapse, including who to contact and wishes around medication.

Flu vaccination

As people with SMI have an increased risk of cardiovascular disease, they should be offered a flu vaccination.

Supporting behaviour change

Physical health checks do not improve the health of people with SMI if the person is not offered any follow-up (Chew Graham, Chitnis, *et al.* 2014). For morbidity and mortality to be reduced, any identified unhealthy behaviour needs to be modified. There is evidence to suggest that people with SMI can work with healthcare professionals to learn how to make lifestyle adjustments (Campion, Francis, *et al.* 2005, Alvarez-Jimenez, Hetrick, *et al.* 2008).

Recently, a randomised controlled trial of primary care nurses and healthcare assistants supporting people with SMI to change their behaviour, found appointments were well attended and there were fewer inpatient admissions (Osborn, Burton, *et al.* 2019). Structured group education alone is not clinically effective in this group (Holt, Gossage-Worrall, *et al.* 2018) so people referred to groups such as weight management may require additional support to ensure attendance and engagement. The behaviour change approaches described in Chapter 2 are applicable to this group.

Summary

Healthcare professionals in primary care are responsible for carrying out physical health checks for people with SMI. Making practical changes when arranging appointments will make it easier for them to attend. To improve the health of people with SMI and decrease their risk of early mortality, they need support from healthcare professionals to help them change their behaviour.

Vignette

Brian is nineteen years old. He was diagnosed with schizophrenia six months ago. He is responding well to his treatment with olanzapine. Since diagnosis he has gained nearly 2 stone and feels very tired all the time. He does not exercise regularly and eats lots of takeaway meals.

How should the healthcare professional support Brian to reduce his health risks?

Reflective questions

- From the perspective of a person with SMI, how accessible are the health checks in your practice?
- What extra support does your practice team provide, to assist people with SMI to change unhealthy behaviour?
- What else could be done in your primary care centre to improve the physical health of people with SMI?

References

Alvarez-Jimenez, M., Hetrick, S., González-Blanch, C. *et al.* (2008). Non-pharmacological management of antipsychotic-induced weight gain: systematic review and meta-analysis of randomised controlled trials. *The British Journal of Psychiatry: The Journal of Mental Science.* **193**, 101–107.

Barber, S. & Thornicroft, G. (2018). Reducing the mortality gap in people with severe mental disorders: the role of lifestyle psychosocial interventions. *Frontiers in Psychiatry.* **9**, 463. doi.org/10.3389/fpsyt.2018.00463

Burgess, C., Wright, A., Forster, A. *et al.* (2015). Influences on individuals' decisions to take up the offer of a health check: a qualitative study. *Health Expectations.* **18**, 2437–48. http://dx.doi.org/10.1111/hex.12212 (Last accessed 30.8.2021).

Bushe, C., Taylor, M. & Haukka, J. (2010). Mortality in schizophrenia: a measurable clinical endpoint. *Journal of Psychopharmacology.* **24** (4_supplement), 17–25.

Camilloni, L., Ferroni, E., Cendales, B. *et al.* (2013). Methods to increase participation in organised screening programs: a systematic review. *BMC Public Health.* **13**, 464. http://dx.doi.org/10.1186/1471-2458-13-464 (Last accessed 30.8.2021).

Campion, G., Francis, V., Preston, A. *et al.* (2005). Health behaviour and motivation to change. *Journal of Psychiatric and Mental Health Nursing.* **25**, 12–15.

Chew Graham, C., Chitnis, A., Turner, P. *et al.* (2014). Why all GPs should be bothered about Billy. *British Journal of General Practice.* **64** (618), 15.

Equality Act (2010). When a mental health condition becomes a disability. https://www.gov.uk/when-mental-health-condition-becomes-disability (Last accessed 30.8.2021).

Dagani, J., Baldessarini, R., Signorini, G. *et al.* (2019). The age of onset of bipolar disorders. In: G. de Girolamo, P. McGorry & N. Sartorius (eds) *Age of Onset of Mental Disorders.* Switzerland: Springer International Publishing.

De Hert, M., Correll, C., Bobes, J., *et al.* (2011). Physical illness in patients with severe mental disorders. I. Prevalence, impact of medications and disparities in health care. *World Psychiatry.* **10**, 52–77.

Drake, R., Addington, J., Viswanathan, A. *et al.* (2016). How age and gender predict illness course in a first episode nonaffective psychosis cohort. *Journal of Clinical Psychiatry.* **77** (3), 283–289.

Firth, J., Siddiqi, N., Koyanagi, A. *et al.* (2019). The Lancet Psychiatry Commission: a blueprint for protecting physical health in people with mental illness. *The Lancet Psychiatry.* **6** (8), 675–712.

Gidlow, C., Ellis, N., Riley, V. *et al.* (2019). Randomised controlled trial comparing uptake of NHS Health Check in response to standard letters, risk-personalised letters and telephone invitations. *BMC Public Health.* **19** (224). https://doi.org/10.1186/s12889-019-6540-8 (Last accessed 30.8.2021).

Hardy, S. (2013). Physical health checks for people with severe mental illness. *Primary Healthcare.* **23** (10), 24–26.

Hardy, S. (2017). *Tier 3 Mental Health and Wellbeing training for primary care nurses: Behaviour change.* London: Health Education England.

Hardy, S., Deane, K. & Gray, R. (2013). The Northampton Physical Health and Wellbeing Project: The views of patients with severe mental illness regarding their physical health check. *Mental Health in Family Medicine.* **9** (4), 233–240.

Hardy, S. & Gray, R. (2012). Is the use of an invitation letter effective in prompting patients with severe mental illness to attend a primary care physical health check? *Primary Health Care Research & Development.* **13** (4), 347–352.

Hayes, J., Marston, L., Walters, K. *et al.* (2017). Mortality gap for people with bipolar disorder and schizophrenia: UK-based cohort study 2000–2014. *The British Journal of Psychiatry.* **211** (3), 175-181.

Holt, R., Gossage-Worrall, R., Hind, D. *et al.* (2018). Structured lifestyle education for people with schizophrenia, schizoaffective disorder and first-episode psychosis (STEPWISE): randomised controlled trial. *The British Journal of Psychiatry.* doi: 10.1192/bjp.2018.167.

Hotopf, M. & McCracken, L. (2014). Physical health in mental illness. In: S.C. Davies (ed.) *Annual Report of the Chief Medical Officer 2013, Public Mental Health Priorities: Investing in the Evidence.* London: Department of Health.

Kisely, S., Crowe, E. & Lawrence, D. (2013). Cancer-related mortality in people with mental illness. *JAMA Psychiatry.* **70** (2), 209–217.

Liu, N., Daumit, G., Dua, T. *et al.* (2017). Excess mortality in persons with severe mental disorders: a multilevel intervention framework and priorities for clinical practice, policy and research agendas. *World Psychiatry.* **16** (1), 30–40.

Marmot, M. (2010). *Fair Society, Healthy Lives, The Marmot Review, Executive Summary.* http://www.instituteofhealthequity.org/resources-reports/fair-society-healthy-lives-the-marmot-review/fair-society-healthy-lives-exec-summary-pdf.pdf (Last accessed 30.8.2021).

McClean, S., Booth, A., Gee, M. *et al.* (2016). Appointment reminder systems are effective but not optimal: results of a systematic review and evidence synthesis employing realist principles. *Patient Preference and Adherence.* **10**, 479–499.

McDermott, L., Wright, A., Cornelius, V. *et al.* (2016). Enhanced invitation methods and uptake of health checks in primary care: randomised controlled trial and cohort study using electronic health records. *Health Technology Assessment.* **20** (84). http://eprints.lse.ac.uk/67916/ (Last accessed 30.8.2021).

McManus, S., Bebbington, P., Jenkins, R. *et al.* (2016). *Mental health and wellbeing in England: Adult Psychiatric Morbidity Survey 2014.* content.digital.nhs.uk (Last accessed 30.8.2021).

MHFA England (2019). Mental Health Statistics. https://mhfaengland.org/mhfa-centre/research-and-evaluation/mental-health-statistics/#psychosis-and-schizophrenia (Last accessed 30.8.2021).

Mitchell, A., Hardy, S. & Shiers D. (2017). Parity of esteem: addressing the inequalities in mental health care as compared with physical health care. *British Journal of Psychiatric Advances.* **23** (3), 196–205.

Mitchell, A., Vancampfort, D., Sweers, K. *et al.* (2013). Prevalence of metabolic syndrome and metabolic abnormalities in schizophrenia and related disorders: a systematic review and meta-analysis. *Schizophrenia Bulletin.* **39**, 306–318.

Nash, M. (2013). Diagnostic overshadowing: a potential barrier to physical health care for mental health service users. *Journal of Mental Health Nursing.* **17** (4), 22–26.

National Institute for Health and Care Excellence (NICE) (2014a). Psychosis and schizophrenia in adults: treatment and management. http://www.nice.org.uk/guidance/cg178/resources/guidance-psychosis-and-schizophrenia-in-adults-treatment-and-management-pdf (Last accessed 30.8.2021).

National Institute of Health and Care Excellence (NICE) (2014b). Bipolar disorder: the assessment and management of bipolar disorder in adults, children and young people in primary and secondary care. http://www.nice.org.uk/guidance/cg185/resources/guidance-bipolar-disorder-the-assessment-and-management-of-bipolar-disorder-in-adults-children-and-young-people-in-primary-and-secondary-care-pdf (Last accessed 30.8.2021).

Norman, P. & Conner, M. (1993). The role of social cognition models in predicting attendance at health checks. *Psychology & Health.* **8**, 447–462.

Olfson, M., Gerhard, T., Huang, C. *et al.* (2015). Premature mortality among adults with schizophrenia in the United States. *JAMA Psychiatry.* **72**, 1172–1181.

Osborn, D., Burton, A., Walters, K. *et al.* (2019). Primary care management of cardiovascular risk for people with severe mental illnesses: the Primrose research programme including cluster RCT. *Programme Grants for Applied Research.* **7** (2).

Perron, N., Dao, M., Kossovsky, M., *et al.* (2010). Reduction of missed appointments at an urban primary care clinic: a randomised controlled study. *BMC Family Practice.* **11**, 79.

Pew Research Center (2019). *Smartphone Ownership Is Growing Rapidly Around the World, but Not Always Equally.* https://www.pewresearch.org/global/2019/02/05/smartphone-ownership-is-growing-rapidly-around-the-world-but-not-always-equally/ (Last accessed 30.8.2021).

Prochaska, J., Norcross, J. & Diclemente, C. (1994). *Changing for Good.* New York: Avon Books.

Public Health England (PHE) (2020). *Vaping in England: an evidence update including mental health and pregnancy, March 2020.* https://assets.publishing.service.gov.uk/government/uploads/system/uploads/attachment_data/file/869401/Vaping_in_England_evidence_update_March_2020.pdf (Last accessed 30.8.2021).

Reda, S. & Makhoul S. (2001). Prompts to encourage appointment attendance for people with serious mental illness. *Cochrane Database Systematic Review.* (2) CD002085.

Sallis, A., Sherlock, J., Bonus, A. *et al*. (2019). Pre-notification and reminder SMS text messages with behaviourally informed invitation letters to improve uptake of NHS Health Checks: a factorial randomised controlled trial. *BMC Public Health*. **19**, 1162. https://doi.org/10.1186/s12889-019-7476-8 (Last accessed 30.8.2021).

Torniainen, M., Mittendorfer-Rutz, E., Tanskanen, A. *et al*. (2015). Antipsychotic treatment and mortality in schizophrenia. *Schizophrenia Bulletin*. **41**, 656–663.

Waddell, L. & Taylor M. (2008). A new self-rating scale for detecting atypical or second generation antipsychotic side effects. *Journal of Psychopharmacology*. **22** (3), 238–243.

Woodhead, C., Ashworth, M., Broadbent, M. *et al*. (2016). Cardiovascular disease treatment among patients with severe mental illness: a data linkage study between primary and secondary care. *British Journal of General Practice*. **66**, e374–81.

Wu, C., Chang, C., Hayes, R. *et al*. (2012). Clinical risk assessment rating and all-cause mortality in secondary mental healthcare: the South London and Maudsley NHS Foundation Trust Biomedical Research Centre (SLAM BRC) Case Register. *Psychological Medicine*. **42**, 1581–1590.

CHAPTER 5

Learning disability

Learning outcomes

By the end of this chapter the reader will:

- Understand what is meant by learning disability
- Be aware of physical health issues in people with a learning disability
- Know how to communicate with a person with a learning disability
- Consider how to make reasonable adjustments
- Know how to monitor physical health in learning disability
- Understand how to support healthy behaviour in people with a learning disability

Introduction

A learning disability should not be confused with a learning difficulty (such as dyslexia) which does not affect intellect. As defined by the Department of Health (2001), a learning disability includes a significantly reduced ability to understand new or complex information, to learn new skills (impaired intelligence), with a reduced ability to cope independently (impaired social functioning). These characteristics will have started before adulthood, and will have a lasting effect on development.

A simpler definition is provided by the learning disability charity Mencap (2020). They describe a learning disability as reduced intellectual ability and difficulty with everyday activities – for example, household tasks, socialising or managing money, which affects someone for their whole life. They go on to explain that people with a learning disability tend to take longer to learn, and may need support to develop new skills, understand complicated information and interact with others.

There are approximately 1.5 million people (more than 2% of the population) with a learning disability in the UK (Office for National Statistics 2019), of which 1.2 million are in England (Public Health England 2016).

Causes of learning disability

A learning disability happens when the brain is still developing, so it can occur before, during or soon after birth:

- Before birth – due to accident or illness in pregnancy; central nervous system (the brain and spinal cord) being impaired during development; or genetic causes

- During birth – due to oxygen deprivation; trauma to the head; or premature birth
- After birth – due to early childhood illnesses; or accidents or seizures.

Some conditions are not a learning disability, but they are associated with learning disability. These are cerebral palsy, William's syndrome, Down's syndrome, fragile X syndrome, autism, and global development delay.

William's syndrome

William's syndrome is a rare (but not hereditary) genetic condition which affects one in 18,000 people in the UK (Mencap 2020). People with William's syndrome usually have the same distinctive facial characteristics, which include a wide mouth, rounded cheeks, and widely spaced teeth. They are often very talkative and can be overly friendly. Anxiety and depression are commonly experienced by this group.

Down's syndrome

Down's syndrome is caused when the person is born with an extra copy of their 21st chromosome. It is not a hereditary condition. People with Down's syndrome will usually have a degree of learning disability and characteristic physical features. Some may have heart problems, visual impairment, or hearing difficulties.

Fragile X syndrome

Fragile X is the most common inherited cause of learning disability. People with this syndrome usually have a long narrow face with prominent jawbones and ears. It is a genetic condition which causes a variety of problems with language, behaviour, emotions, attention, and social interaction. Most boys with Fragile X syndrome will have a learning disability but only one-third of girls will. Common behaviours observed in those with this condition include avoiding eye contact, and hand flapping or hand biting. They often feel anxious in social situations, tend to be very shy, and prefer familiar routines.

Autism

Autism is often referred to as autism spectrum disorder (ASD). It may affect the person's interactions with others in a social situation, ability to communicate with others, and experience of the world around them. Approximately half of people with autism have a learning disability.

Global development delay

Global development delay (GDD) is the term used when a child does not reach expected development milestones – for example, walking, talking, learning, and interacting with others.

For some, GDD is short-term and can be treated with support or therapy, but for others it is significant and is an indication of a learning disability.

How a person is affected by a learning disability

A person's learning disability may be mild, moderate, severe or profound – and they will usually require some level of help. Those with a mild learning disability may be able to interact well with others and cope with some everyday tasks, whereas people with a severe learning disability or profound and multiple learning disability (PMLD) will need care and support with communication, mobility and personal care. This may be provided by paid carers or support workers or by members of their family (National Guideline Alliance UK 2016).

People with a learning disability are more likely to display challenging behaviour than the rest of the population. This may be because they are having difficulty communicating, or they are in pain or discomfort, or struggling with their mental health. They are also more likely to have a mental health problem. A large study in the UK, which included 1,023 adults with learning disabilities, found that 28.3% had current mental health difficulties if those with problem behaviours were excluded, and 40.9% when those with problem behaviours were included (Cooper, Smiley, *et al.* 2007). This compares with 19.7% in the general population (Evans, Macrory & Randall 2016). Anxiety disorders, depression, schizophrenia and dementia are commonly experienced by people with learning disabilities (Blair 2019, NHS England and NHS Improvement 2020).

Physical health issues in people with a learning disability

People with a learning disability are more likely to suffer from physical health problems, such as gastrointestinal cancers, including those of the oesophagus, stomach and gall bladder; coronary heart disease; dental problems and poor oral hygiene; diabetes; epilepsy; gastrointestinal problems; obesity; respiratory disease; visual and auditory impairment; and swallowing and eating problems (Blair 2019).

Though the life expectancy of people with learning disabilities is increasing, it is on average 20 years less in this group than in the general population (O'Leary, Cooper & Hughes-McCormack 2018). The most common causes of death recorded in England in order are: pneumonia, aspiration pneumonia, sepsis, dementia, cardiovascular disease, and epilepsy (NHS England and NHS Improvement 2020).

A confidential enquiry found that some of the reasons for increased mortality amongst those with a learning disability are related to preventable causes and could be reduced through access to national screening programmes or better-quality healthcare (Heslop, Blair, *et al.* 2013). The authors report that 38% of people with a learning disability died from an avoidable cause, compared to 9% of people without a learning disability. Perera, Audi, *et al.* (2019) explain that studies have shown people with a learning disability get suboptimal care and they offer some reasons for this:

- They do not present to their GPs, so treatable conditions are not identified early, or ever.
- They may receive little or no guidance on improving their health through actions such as nutrition and exercise.
- Diagnostic overshadowing – this is when symptoms caused by physical or mental health problems are wrongly attributed to the person's learning disability, leading to delayed diagnosis and treatment (Ali, Scior, *et al.* 2013).

- They may be less likely to receive appropriate investigations, screening and treatment than people in the general population. Statistics compiled by NHS Digital (2019) showed that in 2017/18, less screening was carried out in the eligible learning disability population than in the eligible general public: 52.5% versus 68% for breast cancer; 31.2% versus 73.2% for cervical cancer; and 77.8% versus 83.7% for colorectal cancer.

Furthermore, there is a much higher rate of drugs prescribed for mental health problems (antipsychotics, antidepressants, drugs used in mania and hypomania, anxiolytics and hypnotics) among people with learning disabilities than in the general population (Glover, Williams, *et al.* 2015). These drugs can contribute to the development of cardiovascular disease, diabetes and obesity (Torniainen, Mittendorfer-Rutz, *et al.* 2015, Mitchell, Vancampfort, *et al.* 2013). In most cases there is no clear justification for prescribing these drugs and they are often used for long periods without adequate review (NICE 2017).

Communicating with a person with a learning disability

The same approach used when communicating with the general population (active listening, open questions, relaxed body posture, calm tone of voice, reflection to ensure mutual understanding) should be used with a person with a learning disability. Mencap (2020) offer some further suggestions:
- Allow more time to prevent rushing
- Use accessible language
- Avoid jargon and long words
- Talk clearly
- Use communication tools such as real objects, pictures or photographs, or draw
- Observe the person's facial expressions and gestures
- Ask parents or carers for their help
- Use gestures and facial expressions.

Some people with a learning disability communicate using Makaton. This is a unique language programme that uses symbols, signs and speech. It can be personalised and used at the level most suitable for the individual. The Makaton charity provide lots of information on their website (Makaton 2021).

Information documents written in an accessible style are helpful to use with people with a learning disability, and some are available free of charge. One source is the EasyRead website (2021). There are other helpful resources about the annual health check for people with learning disabilities, their families and for professionals involved in their care on the National Development Team for Inclusion's website (NDTi 2021). And NHS England provide a template invitation letter on their website (NHS England 2021).

Making reasonable adjustments

Researchers have reported the reasons that people with a learning disability do not get appropriate healthcare (Heslop, Blair *et al.* 2013, Tuffrey-Wijne, Giatras *et al.* 2013, Allerton & Emerson 2012). These include:

- They are not recognised as having a learning disability
- Care providers have a poor understanding of learning disability or lack confidence
- Ill health goes unrecognised
- Correct diagnosis not made
- Different care providers not communicating
- Carers not permitted to be involved
- Inadequate follow-up care.

People with learning disabilities are entitled to reasonable adjustments under the Equality Act (2010) to minimise the disadvantages they face when using services. Healthcare professionals have a legal duty to provide these reasonable adjustments (Public Health England 2016).

It is helpful if healthcare professionals in primary care carry out some preparatory work, such as finding out what would help each person with a learning disability best manage their visit. Other adjustments could include (Norman 2017):

- Using Easy Read materials to communicate and check understanding
- Providing longer appointments
- Accommodating those who are particularly anxious or agitated by giving them an early appointment at the beginning of a session or a late appointment when the clinic is quieter.

Monitoring physical health in people with a learning disability

National guidance for people with learning disabilities recommends an annual health check for those aged 14 years or over to identify undetected health conditions early, ensure the appropriateness of ongoing treatments, establish trust and support continuity of care (NICE 2015, 2019).

People with a learning disability are identified in primary care through the Quality and Outcome Framework (QOF) disease registers. The most recent audit of these registers showed that only about 25% of people in England with a learning disability were recorded on the Learning Disability QOF register (Public Health England 2016). These registers need to be accurate to ensure that these individuals are offered their annual health check. Although the number of people with a learning disability receiving a health check is increasing, only 55.1% of those on the register had one in 2017–18, and only 44.9% received a flu immunisation in the same year (NHS Digital 2019).

The health check should involve personalised care planning to manage comorbidities, reduce unnecessary hospitalisations, promote health positively and reduce premature mortality (NHS England

and NHS Improvement 2020). It should also include a medication review, with a view to implementing planned supervised dose reduction and stopping of inappropriate psychotropic drugs (NHS England 2015).

The Royal College of General Practitioners (RCGP) recommends using the Welsh Health Check template for adults with a learning disability (Kerr, Jones & Hoghton 2016) which is designed to support primary care doctors and nurses to provide a systemic physical health check including physical examination, medical review and health check action plan. It takes approximately an hour to complete. It has been reproduced below but is also freely available from the RCGP website (RCGP 2020). Some primary care centres may have this as a template on their computer system.

Welsh Health Check for Adults with a Learning Disability

Date:	
Name:	
Marital status:	Ethnic origin:
Date of birth:	Sex:
Address: Tel:	
Next of kin: Tel:	
Principal carer: Tel:	

KEY HEALTH AND SOCIAL CARE CONTACTS:		
Consent to share the review with the carer?	**Yes**	**No**
Consent to share the review with other named relevant professionals?	**Yes**	**No**
Names of other individuals to whom the review should be sent:		

This is a good time to ask the carer and the person with a learning disability if they have any specific concerns or issues they wish to discuss whilst performing the health check.

Weight (kg/stone):	Height (metres/feet):
Blood pressure:	Urine analysis:
Smoke (cigarettes per day):	Alcohol (units per week):

Body Mass Index (weight in kg/height in m^2):

Cholesterol has been performed if indicated:	Random Blood Glucose if indicated:

Date of last ECG:

(risk is highest for antipsychotics such as Haloperidol/older antipsychotics, Quetiapine or tricyclic antidepressants)

Immunisation

People with learning disability should have the same regimes as others and the same contraindications apply. A high risk of hepatitis 'b' has been seen in individuals with learning disability.

Has the patient completed a full course of currently recommended vaccinations?	**Yes**	**No**
If No, has the patient been offered the recommended top-up vaccinations?	**Yes**	**No**
Is the patient included in the annual influenza vaccination programme?	**Yes**	**No**
Patient declined/contraindicated	**Yes**	

Screening uptake

Where screening cannot be performed due to refusal, it can be helpful for the community learning disability team to support the individual through the procedures.

Cervical cytology - People with a learning disability have the same indications for cervical cytology as others. **Note:** Smear could be declined by patient.

Is a smear indicated?	**Yes**	**No**

If yes, when was last smear?	
When is next smear due?	**Date:**
Patient declined	**Yes**

Mammography uptake
This should be arranged in line with national screening programme and as per local practice.

Is mammography indicated and has it been offered?	**Yes**	**No**
Performed?	**Yes**	**No**
Declined?	**Yes**	**No**

Bowel cancer uptake
This should be arranged in line with national screening programme and as per local practice.

Indicated and offered?	**Yes**	**No**
Performed?	**Yes**	**No**
Declined?	**Yes**	**No**

Aortic aneurysm uptake
This should be arranged in line with national screening programme and as per local practice.

Indicated and offered?	**Yes**	**No**
Performed?	**Yes**	**No**
Declined?	**Yes**	**No**

Chronic illness

Does your patient suffer from any chronic illness?	**Yes**	**No**
If yes, please specify:		

SYSTEMS ENQUIRY

Respiratory

Be especially concerned if the person has frequent chest infections as these can indicate that swallowing is impaired and referral is needed.

Number of chest infections in previous 12 months:

Persistent cough	Yes	No
Haemoptysis	Yes	No
Abnormal sputum	Yes	No
Wheeze	Yes	No
Dyspnoea	Yes	No

Cardiovascular system

Chest pain	Yes	No
Swelling of ankles	Yes	No
Palpitations	Yes	No
Paroxysmal nocturnal dyspnoea	Yes	No
Cyanosis	Yes	No

Abdominal

Be aware of possibility of unrecognised reflux oesophagitis as a cause of weight loss, sleep disturbance or dyspepsia.

Constipation	Yes	No
Weight loss	Yes	No
Diarrhoea	Yes	No
Dyspepsia	Yes	No
Melaena	Yes	No
Rectal bleeding	Yes	No
Faecal incontinence	Yes	No
Feeding problems	Yes	No

Central nervous system – for Epilepsy, see below

Faints	**Yes**	**No**
Parasthesia	**Yes**	**No**
Weakness	**Yes**	**No**

Genito-urinary

Dysuria	**Yes**	**No**
Frequency	**Yes**	**No**
Haematuria	**Yes**	**No**
Urinary incontinence	**Yes**	**No**
If Yes, has mid-stream urine (MSU) been done	**Yes**	**No**
Have other investigations been considered?	**Yes**	**No**

Gynaecological

Dysmenorrhoea	**Yes**	**No**
Inter-menstrual bleeding	**Yes**	**No**
Vaginal discharge	**Yes**	**No**
Is patient post-menopausal?	**Yes**	**No**
Contraceptives needed	**Yes**	**No**
Used **Note:** Oral, intra-uterine device, depot, transdermal, subcutaneous, diaphragm, contraceptive sponge, no contraception	**Yes**	**No**
Other **Note:** e.g. Pre-menstrual treatment, pregnancy		

Epilepsy **Note:** Consider specialist review if no review has been done in last 3 years	**Yes**	**No**
Date of last specialist appointment: Less than 3 years ago	**Yes**	**No**

More than 3 years ago		Yes		No	
Type of fit:					
Focal seizures: simple partial, complex partial or secondary generalised		Yes		No	
Generalised seizures: absence seizures, myoclonic, clonic, tonic, tonic-clonic or atonic		Yes		No	
Unclassified seizures		Yes		No	
Frequency of seizures (fits/month)					
Over the last year have the fits:	**Worsened?**		**Remained the same?**		**Improved?**
Anti-epileptic medication					
Name, dose/frequency levels (if indicated)					
Side effects observed in the patient					

Behavioural and mental ill health

Note: Behavioural disturbance in people with a learning disability is often an indicator of some other morbidity. For this reason, it is important to record it, as it can point to other morbidities.

The presence of behavioural or emotional change when physical illness has been excluded warrants referral to learning disability services.

When concerned about a person with a learning disability, it is always good practice to try and talk to them on their own to see if there are stresses or concerns they don't want to discuss in front of carers.

	Yes	No
Has there been a change in behaviour since the last review, e.g. aggression, self-injury or over-activity?	Yes	No
Are you aware of any risk or change in the level of risk to the patient or others?	Yes	No
If yes, has this been communicated to key health and social care professionals?	Yes	No
Does the person have a recorded mental illness?	Yes	No
If so, is the person on medication for this?	Yes	No

Are there possible signs or concerns over the known mental illness or the possibility of a new condition?	Yes	No

You may consider referral to mental health services to address this.

General appearance

Are there any abnormal physical signs or key negative findings?	Yes	No
If yes, please specify:		

Cardiovascular system

Are there any abnormal physical signs or key negative findings?	Yes	No
If yes, please specify:		
Pulse (beats/min):	Regular	Irregular
Blood pressure:		
Ankle oedema:	Yes	No
Heart sounds (? describe) Murmurs/added sounds	Yes	No
Patient declined	Yes	

Respiratory system

Are there any abnormal physical signs or key negative findings?	Yes	No

If yes, please specify:		
Patient declined	**Yes**	

Abdomen

Are there any abnormal physical signs or key negative findings?	**Yes**	**No**
If yes, please specify:		
Patient declined	**Yes**	**No**

Dermatology

Any signs or symptoms?	**Yes**
Diagnosis:	
Patient declined	**Yes**

Breast

Are you aware of any breast symptoms or signs?	**Yes**	**No**
If yes, please indicate what action has been taken:		
Note: If no, please indicate why (e.g. consent issues):		
Patient declined	**Yes**	

Testes

Has an examination of the testes been performed?	**Yes**	**No**
Patient declined	**Yes**	

Central nervous system

Note: It is often difficult and not relevant to perform a full neurological examination. However, people with a learning disability are particularly prone to abnormalities in vision, hearing and communication – a change in function would suggest that further investigation is necessary.

Presence of vision difficulties

Does the patient appear to have eyesight problems e.g. eye rubbing?	**Yes**	**No**
Normal vision? **Note:** include normal vision corrected with glasses/contact lenses	**Yes**	**No**
Minor visual problem?	**Yes**	**No**
Major visual problem? **Note:** include registered blind	**Yes**	**No**
Is the carer/key worker concerned?	**Yes**	**No**
Recommend the carer takes the patient to an optometrist	**Yes**	**No**
Is there a cataract?	**Yes**	**No**

Presence of hearing difficulties

Normal hearing?	**Yes**	**No**
Minor hearing problem?	**Yes**	**No**
Major hearing problem?	**Yes**	**No**
Is the carer/key worker concerned?	**Yes**	**No**
Does the person wear a hearing aid? **Note:** if no, has the person been fitted for a hearing aid?	**Yes**	**No**
Any wax present?	**Yes**	**No**
Does your patient see an audiologist?	**Yes**	**No**

Other investigations:
- Has the patient ever had a hearing screen?
- For those aged 40 and over, has the patient had a hearing screen within the past 3 years?
- For those with Down's syndrome (regardless of age), has the patient had a hearing assessment within the past 3 years?

Presence of communication difficulties

Does your patient communicate normally?	**Yes**	**No**
Does your patient communicate with aids? **Note:** e.g. writing pad, signing	**Yes**	**No**
Does your patient have a severe communication problem?	**Yes**	**No**
Does your patient see a speech therapist?	**Yes**	**No**
Where communication problems exist, have practice staff been made aware, has the person's medical record been tagged?	**Yes**	**No**

Presence of mobility difficulties

Is your patient fully mobile?	**Yes**	**No**
If no, please specify the nature and severity of mobility loss, such as presence of contractures, e.g. uses a wheelchair, walking stick, walking frame, crutches, splints, surgical boots		
Has there been any change in the patient's mobility and dexterity since the last review?	**Yes**	**No**
If yes, please specify:		

Other investigations

Are any further investigations necessary?	**Yes**	**No**
If yes, please indicate:		

Syndrome-specific check

Note: Certain syndromes that cause learning disabilities are associated with increased morbidity. For this reason, it is important to record:

Is the cause of learning disability known?	**Yes**	**No**
If yes, what is it?		
Has the patient had a genetic investigation?	**Yes**	**No**
Result?		
If your patient has Down's syndrome, they should have a yearly thyroid profile.		
Has this been done?	**Yes**	**No**
If your patient has Down's syndrome, please ask family members, carers or care workers (as appropriate) about any changes that might suggest the need for an assessment of dementia, such as:		
Any change in the person's behaviour?	**Yes**	**No**
Any loss of skills (including self-care)?	**Yes**	**No**
A need for more prompting in the past few months?	**Yes**	**No**

Have a low threshold for excluding concurrent physical morbidity and/or referral to mental health services.

Medication review

Is the person taking antipsychotic medication without a recorded mental health illness?	**Yes**	**No**
Could any of the psychotropic medication be reduced or stopped?	**Yes**	**No**

Drug	Dose	Side effects	Levels (if indicated)

Please list the key findings from the medication review:

Actions

Please list the actions that have arisen as a result of the medication review and indicate how these have been dealt with:

Every year the patient should have a review by a dental practitioner – has this been done?	Yes	No
Every year the patient should have a review by an optometrist – has this been done?	Yes	No
Has a summary letter with appropriate responses been sent to the patient or carer?	**Yes**	**No**
Has a copy of the letter been sent to the community learning disability team if involved?	**Yes**	**No**

Supporting healthy behaviour in people with a learning disability

It is important to remember that people with learning disabilities have the same legal right to make their own choices as everyone else (Norman 2017). A government White Paper found that carers feel strongly that they have a lifelong responsibility for the person and want to be treated as full partners by public agencies (DoH 2001). Both parties need appropriate personalised information and support to enable them to carry out the recommended actions identified in the health check. There is a need for healthcare professionals in primary care to consider how further visits can be organised to accommodate this.

Summary

Healthcare professionals in primary care are responsible for carrying out an annual review for people with a learning disability. Making reasonable adjustments will make it easier for this group to engage with primary healthcare services. To improve the health of people with a learning disability and decrease their risk of early mortality, support needs to be given to carry out the recommended actions identified in the health check.

Vignette

Amanda is 26 years old and lives with her mother. She has Down's syndrome. She goes to a day centre three times a week, which she enjoys. Amanda loves food, particularly cakes. She has a BMI of 33 and she does not drink alcohol or smoke.

How should the healthcare professional support Amanda and her mum to reduce her health risks?

Reflective questions

- From the perspective of a person with a learning disability, how good are the reasonable adjustments made by your primary care centre?
- What extra support is provided by your practice team to assist people with a learning disability to be healthy?
- What else could be done in your primary care centre to improve the care of people with a learning disability?

References

Ali, A., Scior, K., Ratti, V. *et al.* (2013). Discrimination and other barriers to accessing health care: perspectives of patients with mild and moderate intellectual disability and their carers. *PLoS One.* **8** (8), e70855.

Allerton, L. & Emerson, E. (2012). British adults with chronic health conditions or impairments face significant barriers to accessing health services. *Public Health.* **126**, 920–927.

Blair, J. (2019). Common health problems of people with learning disabilities. *British Journal of Family Medicine.* https://www.bjfm.co.uk/blog/common-health-problems-of-people-with-learning-disabilities-blog (Last accessed 1.9.2021).

Cooper, S.-A., Smiley, E., Morrison, J. *et al.* (2007). Prevalence of and associations with mental ill-health in adults with intellectual disabilities. *British Journal of Psychiatry.* **190**, 27–35.

Department of Health (DoH) (2001). *Valuing People: A New Strategy for Learning Disability for the 21st Century.* London: DoH.

EasyRead (2021). http://easyread.info/free-easy-read-resources-accessible/ (Last accessed 1.9.2021).

Equality Act (2010). When a mental health condition becomes a disability. https://www.gov.uk/when-mental-health-condition-becomes-disability (Last accessed 30.8.2021).

Evans, J., Macrory, I. & Randall, C. (2016). *Measuring national well-being: Life in the UK, 2016.* ONS. https://www.ons.gov.uk/peoplepopulationandcommunity/wellbeing/articles/measuringnationalwellbeing/2016#how-good-is-our-health (Last accessed 1.9.2021).

Glover, G., Williams, R., Branford, D. *et al.* (2015). *Prescribing of psychotropic drugs to people with learning disabilities and/or autism by general practitioners in England.* Public Health England.

Heslop, P., Blair, P., Fleming, P. *et al.* (2013). *Confidential inquiry into premature deaths of people with learning disabilities: final report.* Bristol: University of Bristol. https://tinyurl.com/yc9m9n75 (Last accessed 1.9.2021).

Kerr, M., Jones, R., Hoghton, M. *et al.* (2016). *Welsh Health Check for Adults with a Learning Disability and on the Social Services Register – revised 2016.* https://www.choiceforum.org/docs/chc.pdf (Last accessed 1.9.2021).

Makaton Charity (2021). https://www.makaton.org/TMC/About_Makaton/What_is_Makaton.aspx (Last accessed 1.9.2021).

Mencap (2020). *What is a learning disability?* https://www.mencap.org.uk/learning-disability-explained/what-learning-disability?gclid=EAIaIQobChMIo4rv--7o6wIVCrh3Ch0YRwV_EAAYASAAEgKrFvD_BwE (Last accessed 1.9.2021).

Mitchell, A., Vancampfort, D., Sweers, K. *et al.* (2013). Prevalence of metabolic syndrome and metabolic abnormalities in schizophrenia and related disorders: a systematic review and meta-analysis. *Schizophrenia Bulletin.* **39**, 306–18.

National Development Team for inclusion (NDTi) (2021). https://www.ndti.org.uk/resources/useful-tools/health-check-resources (Last accessed 1.9.2021).

National Guideline Alliance (UK) (2016). *Mental Health Problems in People with Learning Disabilities: Prevention, Assessment and Management.* London: NICE.

National Institute for Health and Care Excellence (NICE) (2015). *Learning disability: behaviour that challenges. Quality standard [QS101].* London: NICE.

National Institute for Health and Care Excellence (NICE) (2019). *Learning disability: care and support of people growing older. Quality standard [QS187].* London: NICE.

National Institute for Health and Care Excellence (NICE) (2017). *Psychotropic medicines in people with learning disabilities whose behaviour challenges.* London: NICE.

NHS Digital (2019). *Health and Care of People with Learning Disabilities: 2017-18. Health and Social Care Information Centre.* https://digital.nhs.uk/data-and-information/publications/statistical/health-and-care-of-people-with-learning-disabilities/experimental-statistics-2017-to-2018 (Last accessed 1.9.2021).

NHS England (2015). *Stop Over-Medication of People with a Learning Disability, Autism or Both.* https://www.rcgp.org.uk/-/media/Files/CIRC/Learning-disabilities/STOMP-GP-Prescribing-v17-ONLINE-SELF-PRINT.ashx?la=en (Last accessed 1.9.2021).

NHS England (2021). https://www.england.nhs.uk/wp-content/uploads/2020/06/Letter-what-to-expect-from-your-doctor.pdf (Last accessed 1.9.2021).

NHS England and NHS Improvement (2020). *QOF Quality Improvement domain 2020/21 – Supporting people with learning disabilities.* https://www.england.nhs.uk/wp-content/uploads/2020/02/20-21-qof-qi-supporting-people-with-learning-disabilites.pdf (Last accessed 1.9.2021).

Norman, A. (2017). Providing support to people with learning disabilities in primary care. *Nursing in Practice.* https://www.nursinginpractice.com/clinical/providing-support-to-people-with-learning-disabilities-in-primary-care/ (Last accessed 1.9.2021).

O'Leary, L., Cooper, S.A., Hughes-McCormack, L. (2018). Early death and causes of death of people with intellectual disabilities: A systematic review. *Journal of Applied Research in Intellectual Disabilities.* **31** (3), 325–342.

Office for National Statistics (ONS) (2019). *Estimates of the population for the UK, England and Wales, Scotland and Northern Ireland.* https://www.ons.gov.uk/peoplepopulationandcommunity/populationandmigration/populationestimates/datasets/populationestimatesforukenglandandwalesscotlandandnorthernireland (Last accessed 1.9.2021).

Perera, B., Audi, S., Solomou, S. *et al.* (2019). Mental and physical health conditions in people with intellectual disabilities: Comparing local and national data. *British Journal of Learning Disabilities.* **48** (1), 19–27.

Public Health England (PHE) (2016). *Learning disabilities Observatory. People with learning disabilities in England 2015.* https://www.gov.uk/government/publications/people-with-learning-disabilities-in-england-2015 (Last accessed 1.9.2021).

Royal College of General Practitioners (RCGP) (2020). *Learning disabilities.* https://www.rcgp.org.uk/learningdisabilities/ (Last accessed 1.9.2021).

Torniainen, M., Mittendorfer-Rutz, E., Tanskanen, A. *et al.* (2015). Antipsychotic treatment and mortality in schizophrenia. *Schizophrenia Bulletin.* **41**, 656–663.

Tuffrey-Wijne, I., Giatras, N., Goulding, L. *et al.* (2013). Identifying the factors affecting the implementation of strategies to promote a safer environment for patients with learning disabilities in NHS hospitals: a mixed-methods study. *Health Services and Delivery Research.* **1** (13). https://pubmed.ncbi.nlm.nih.gov/25642531/ (Last accessed 1.9.2021).

CHAPTER 6

Dementia

Learning outcomes

By the end of this chapter the reader will:

- Be aware of the different types of dementia
- Understand how a diagnosis of dementia is made
- Recognise the responsibilities of healthcare professionals in primary care regarding people with dementia

Introduction

Dementia is a term used to describe a range of progressive neurological disorders affecting the brain. The condition is experienced in various ways depending on the type of dementia or the part of the brain affected. The effects of dementia can be physical, emotional and psychological. The person's mental capabilities are disturbed so planning and organising can be difficult. Retaining independence may become a challenge so assistance from friends or relatives is often required.

The symptoms of dementia usually get worse over time. There is no cure for dementia at present, but an early diagnosis can enable attempts to slow down the progression of the disease. An early diagnosis can also allow people with dementia to get the right treatment and support (NHS UK 2020a).

The risk of developing dementia increases with age; therefore, it is most often seen in wealthier countries where people live into very old age. In the UK there are approximately 885,000 people experiencing dementia (Wittenberg, Hu, *et al.* 2019). A report carried out by the Alzheimer's Society (2014) estimated that 42,325 people under the age of 65 years were living with dementia in the UK.

Types of dementia

There are many types of dementia, each characterised by different causes and symptoms. The five most common are: Alzheimer's disease, vascular dementia, Lewy body dementia, frontotemporal dementia, and mixed dementia.

Alzheimer's disease

Around 62% of people in the UK with dementia will have Alzheimer's disease, making it the most common type (Alzheimer's Society 2014). In people with Alzheimer's, 'plaques' and 'tangles' develop in the structures of the brain, leading to the death of brain cells. There is a shortage of certain key neurotransmitters.

Over time, more of the brain is destroyed and symptoms become more severe. Common symptoms of Alzheimer's disease include:

- In the early stages (typically the first few months):
  - o Lapses of memory and problems finding the right words
- In the later stages (typically months to years):
  - o Confusion: frequently forgetting names, places, appointments, and recent events
  - o Mood swings: may be sad or angry, feeling scared and frustrated by their memory problems
  - o Withdrawal and isolation, due either to a loss of confidence or to communication problems.

Vascular dementia

Vascular dementia is the second most common form of this condition, affecting 17% of people in the UK who have dementia (Alzheimer's Society 2014). Vascular dementia is caused by impaired blood flow to the brain, either from narrowing or complete blockage of blood vessels. This deprives cells of nutrients and oxygen, eventually destroying them.

Narrowing of blood vessels is caused by conditions such as diabetes and hypertension. Blockage is usually the result of several small strokes that occur repeatedly over time or it may occur following a major stroke. Because of the different causes of vascular dementia, symptoms may develop suddenly and quickly worsen, or they may develop gradually over many months.

Common symptoms of vascular dementia include:

- Memory loss
- Difficulties with tasks that require concentration and planning
- Depression
- Changes in personality and mood
- Episodes of confusion
- Urinary incontinence
- Poor attention
- Stroke-like symptoms, such as paralysis on one side of the body
- Slow and unsteady gait
- Night-time wandering.

Lewy body dementia

Lewy body dementia is characterised by deposits of the protein alpha-synuclein inside brain cells. These deposits are called Lewy bodies, named after Friedrich H. Lewy, who described them in the early 1900s. There are two types of this dementia: Lewy body dementia which affects 4% of people with dementia; and Parkinson's disease dementia which affects 2% (Alzheimer's Society 2014).

The two can be distinguished by the timing of cognitive and movement symptoms. In Lewy body dementia, cognitive symptoms develop within a year of movement symptoms; and in Parkinson's disease dementia, cognitive symptoms develop more than a year after the onset of movement symptoms. In some people, symptoms develop progressively at a steady rate; in others the decline can be profound and dramatic.

The common symptoms of Lewy body dementia include:

- Memory loss
- Poor attention span
- Episodes of confusion
- Delusions
- Difficulty in planning
- Muscle stiffness
- Slowed movement
- Shaking and trembling of limbs
- Shuffling gait
- Sleep problems
- Loss of facial expression
- Visual hallucinations.

Frontotemporal dementia

Frontotemporal dementia affects 2% of people with dementia in the UK (Alzheimer's Society 2014). It usually occurs in those between 50 and 60 years of age. It is caused by damage to the frontal or temporal lobe of the brain, which controls emotional responses and behaviour. Consequently, many of the initial symptoms of frontotemporal dementia involve changes in emotion, personality and behaviour.

People with this form of dementia may become less sensitive to other people's emotions, which can make them appear selfish and unfeeling. They may become disinhibited, which can lead to inappropriate behaviour – for example, making sexually suggestive gestures in a public place, being rude to others, or making tactless comments.

Other symptoms of frontotemporal dementia include:

- Aggression
- Compulsive behaviour
- Being easily distracted
- Lack of interest in personal hygiene
- Change in personality.

Frontotemporal dementia can also cause problems with language, and people may have problems finding the right words to express themselves. So, they may use many words instead of a few to describe something. For example, they might say, *'a metal tool with a long handle used for digging'* instead of *'a spade'*.

It is important to note that in this form of dementia, the person's memory often remains intact.

Mixed dementia

Around 10% of people with dementia in the UK will have mixed dementia. This means they have two types of dementia. The most common permutation is Alzheimer's disease and vascular dementia. A person with mixed dementia will experience a mixture of the symptoms related to the types of dementia they have. They are more likely to be over the age of 75. Mixed dementia is often not recognised, and the person may be diagnosed as having one type of dementia.

Responsibilities of healthcare professionals

Public Health England (2018) explain that health and care professionals can help individuals by following NHS England's Well Pathway for Dementia (2016). The pathway includes sections on preventing, diagnosing, living, supporting, and dying.

Preventing well

NHS UK (2020b) advises that what is good for the heart is also good for the brain. Therefore, the risk of dementia can be reduced by: eating a healthy balanced diet; maintaining a healthy weight; exercising regularly; keeping alcohol within recommended limits; stopping smoking; keeping blood pressure at a healthy level; treating depression; and tackling loneliness and social isolation. As part of daily contact with individuals, healthcare professionals in primary care can offer this information and support (Public Health England 2018). Additionally, when carrying out an NHS health check, the practitioner should advise those over the age of 65 about the signs and symptoms of dementia and how to lower their risk (NHS UK 2020b).

Diagnosing well

The national guidelines for dementia (NICE 2019) state that healthcare practitioners should investigate reversible causes of cognitive decline, such as delirium, depression, sensory impairment (such as sight or hearing loss) or cognitive impairment from medicines associated with increased anticholinergic burden. It goes on to say that if dementia is still suspected they should be referred to a specialist dementia diagnostic service, but only if they agree. Before referral, the healthcare professional in primary care should carry out (NICE 2018):

- A detailed medical history
- Medication reconciliation to identify any drugs that may impair cognitive functioning
- A full physical examination
- Blood tests (full blood count, calcium, glucose, renal and liver function, thyroid function tests, serum vitamin B12 and folate levels)
- A midstream urine test to rule out infection
- Clinical cognitive assessment using a standardised measure of cognitive functioning:
    - o the 10-point cognitive screener (10-CS)
    - o the 6-item cognitive impairment test (6CIT)

- o   the 6-item screener
- o   the Memory Impairment Screen (MIS)
- o   the Mini-Cog
- o   Test Your Memory (TYM). The 7-Minute Screen

These tools can be found on the Patient.info website (2021).

The specialist dementia diagnostic service will provide:

- A comprehensive assessment
- Confirm diagnosis
- Initiate treatment
- Provide information, advice and support for families and carers
- Signpost patients and carers to social care and voluntary organisations that can provide additional support and services.

Following a dementia diagnosis, a care plan should be drawn up, setting out the care that might be needed by the individual and the people who care for them. This may be developed by the specialist dementia diagnostic service, social services, or the GP, together with the person with dementia and their carer (NHS UK 2018).

The care plan should include:

- How the person can continue activities for as long as possible
- Information about services and how to access them
- Any health conditions that need regular monitoring
- The name of a health or social care person who will coordinate support.

The plan should be reviewed at least once a year.

People with dementia should be given information about advance care planning at diagnosis and at each health and social care review (NICE 2019). Advance care planning enables people to make decisions about their future care before they find it difficult to communicate or lack the capacity to do so. They should be given the opportunity to review and change the plan as the dementia progresses and if their preferences or needs change.

Living well

The healthcare professional should promote health messages to help improve the physical, mental and oral health of people living with dementia and their carers; support them to choose from a range of activities tailored to their preferences to promote wellbeing and use positive language when talking about dementia. This means using words and phrases that empower people, treat them with dignity, respect them as individuals and make them feel valued and included (Alzheimer's Society 2020a). The language should convey that the healthcare professional recognises dementia is not the defining aspect of a person's life and they see the person, not the dementia. The healthcare professional should also consider how the person with dementia may be feeling, use their own words if appropriate, and focus on what they can do (rather than what they cannot).

Terms when talking about dementia

Focus	Helpful terms	Detrimental terms
Dementia	<ul><li>Dementia (a condition), Alzheimer's disease and other types of dementia</li><li>A form of dementia</li><li>A type of dementia</li><li>Symptoms of dementia</li><li>Young-onset dementia</li></ul>	<ul><li>Dementia (a disease)</li><li>Dementing illness</li><li>Demented</li><li>Affliction</li><li>Senile dementia</li><li>Senility</li></ul>
People living with dementia	<ul><li>A person (or people) with dementia</li><li>A person (or people) living with dementia</li><li>A person (or people) with a diagnosis of dementia</li></ul>	<ul><li>Sufferer</li><li>Suffer from</li><li>Afflicted</li><li>Victim</li><li>Demented patient (when used outside the medical context)</li><li>Not all there</li><li>Lost their mind</li><li>Derogatory slang expressions – for example, delightfully dotty, doolally, away with the fairies</li></ul>
People with dementia under 65	<ul><li>Young-onset dementia</li><li>Working-age dementia</li><li>Early-onset dementia</li></ul>	<ul><li>Pre-senile dementia</li></ul>
The symptoms of dementia	**Describe the symptom itself – for example:**<ul><li>Memory loss</li><li>Difficulty communicating</li><li>Changes in behaviour</li></ul>**Expressions of unmet need:**<ul><li>Challenging behaviours</li><li>Behaviours that challenge</li><li>Behavioural and psychological symptoms (in a clinical context)</li></ul>	<ul><li>Wanderer</li><li>Shouter</li><li>Wandering</li><li>Difficult behaviours</li><li>Being difficult</li></ul>

The impact of dementia	<ul><li>Challenging</li><li>Disabling</li><li>Life-changing</li><li>Stressful</li></ul>	<ul><li>Hopeless</li><li>Unbearable</li><li>Impossible</li><li>Tragic</li></ul>
People caring for a person with dementia	<ul><li>Caring for a person with dementia</li><li>Supporting a person with dementia</li></ul>	<ul><li>Living with dementia</li></ul>
The act of providing care for a person with dementia	<ul><li>Caring</li><li>Supporting/helping the person to eat/dress/go to the toilet</li></ul>	<ul><li>Sitting service</li><li>Sitter</li><li>Feeding</li><li>Dressing</li><li>Toileting</li><li>Burden (for an individual)</li></ul>

Adapted from Alzheimer's Society (2020a).

Supporting well

Healthcare professionals should involve people with dementia and their carers in all care and treatment planning, making it personal (Public Health England 2018). When people living with dementia or their carers have a primary care appointment, they should be assessed for any emerging dementia-related needs and asked if they need any more support (NICE 2018).

Practitioners in primary care can encourage people with dementia to participate in any activities or therapies they have been offered and check concordance with any medication prescribed for dementia. The activities may include group cognitive stimulation therapy, group reminiscence therapy, cognitive rehabilitation or occupational therapy, and non-medical interventions tailored to the person's preferences, skills, and abilities (NICE 2018).

Medication that may be prescribed for dementia includes the three acetylcholinesterase (AChE) inhibitors (donepezil, galantamine and rivastigmine) or memantine. Antipsychotics may be prescribed for people living with dementia who are at risk of harming themselves or others, or experiencing agitation, hallucinations or delusions that are causing them severe distress.

People with dementia should be invited to primary care for an annual review of their care plan (NICE 2019). If they do not already have a care plan or an advanced care plan in place, primary care practitioners are expected to help them develop one (BMA 2019). The review should address the following key issues:

- An appropriate physical, mental health and social review for the person
- A record of their wishes for the future
- Communication and co-ordination arrangements with secondary care (if applicable)
- Identification of the person's carer(s)

- o Gain permission to allow the practice to speak directly to the carer(s)
- o Offer details of support services available
- o Include the carer in the care plan or advanced care plan discussions
- o Discuss the impact of caring on the caregiver
- o Offer the carer a health check. If they are registered at a different practice, inform them that they can seek advice from their own practice.
- Assessment of any behavioural changes caused by:
  - o Concurrent physical conditions (e.g. joint pain or inter-current infections)
  - o New appearance of features inherent in the disorder (e.g. wandering) and delusions or hallucinations due to the dementia or as a result of caring behaviour (e.g. being dressed by a carer).
- Consider depression as it is more common in patients with dementia than in those without
- Provide relevant information about the diagnosis and sources of help and support
- As the illness progresses, the review may focus more on issues such as respite care.

The organisation should make adaptations to support a dementia-friendly environment (Public Health England 2018). The Alzheimer's Society (Alzheimer's Society 2020b) have produced a checklist to highlight the adaptations that will make a building as dementia-friendly and inclusive as possible. This includes:

- Having a quiet space available for someone who might be feeling anxious or confused
- Signage should be:
  - o Clear, in bold face, with good contrast between text and background and a contrast between the sign and the surface it is mounted on, to allow the person to recognise it as a sign
  - o Fixed to the door it refers to
  - o At eye level and well-lit
  - o Representational (not abstract images or icons)
  - o Placed at key decision points for someone who is in the building/area for the first time.
- Lighting – entrances should be well-lit and make as much use of natural light as possible. Bright light or deep shadows should be avoided.
- Flooring – should not be highly reflective, slippery or have bold patterned carpets. Steps should be avoided if possible.
- Toilets should be unisex. Toilet seats that are of a contrasting colour to the walls and rest of the toilet are easier to see if someone has visual problems. A 'Way Out' sign in the toilet should be used to clearly mark the exit.
- Seating should look like seating.
- Navigation – people with dementia use 'landmarks' to navigate their way around, both inside and outside. The more attractive and interesting the landmark (e.g. a painting, or a plant), the easier it is to use it as a landmark.

One outpatient department put up historical photographs and found that this prompted discussion based on people's memories (DoH 2015).

Dying well

Advance care plans for people with dementia should include choices about their death (NICE 2019):

- Wishes, preferences, beliefs and values regarding future care
- Decisions to refuse treatment
- Preferences regarding place of care and place of death
- Cultural or religious preferences or practices.

Summary

Early diagnosis of dementia is essential to try to decelerate the progression of the disease and to help the people get the right treatment and support. An annual review of the person's care plan is the responsibility of primary care practitioners and is key to ensuring that people with dementia and their carers get the information, support, care and treatment required for the effective management of this condition.

Vignette

Douglas is 56 years old and has frontotemporal dementia. He has come for an annual review with his wife Jenny. The healthcare professional notices that Jenny looks tired and unkempt and she is very quiet. She is usually very cheerful and smart.

How should the healthcare professional deal with this situation?

Reflective questions

- Consider how well you and your colleagues take action to prevent dementia.
- What extra support is provided by your practice team to help people with dementia get the best out of their experience in the practice?
- What else could be done in your primary care setting to improve care of people with dementia and their carers?

References

Alzheimer's Society (2014). *Dementia UK update.* https://www.alzheimers.org.uk/sites/default/files/migrate/downloads/dementia_uk_update.pdf (Last accessed 2.9.2021).

Alzheimer's Society (2020a). *Positive language.* https://www.alzheimers.org.uk/sites/default/files/2018-09/Positive%20language%20guide_0.pdf (Last accessed 2.9.2021).

Alzheimer's Society (2020b). *Dementia-friendly environment checklist.* https://www.alzheimers.org.uk/get-involved/dementia-friendly-communities/organisations/dementia-friendly-environment-checklist (Last accessed 2.9.2021).

British Medical Association (BMA) (2019). 2019/20 *General Medical Services (GMS) contract Quality and Outcomes Framework (QOF).* https://www.england.nhs.uk/wp-content/uploads/2019/05/gms-contract-qof-guidance-april-2019.pdf (Last accessed 2.9.2021).

Department of Health (DoH) (2015). Health Building Note 08-02 Dementia-friendly Health and Social Care Environments. https://assets.publishing.service.gov.uk/government/uploads/system/uploads/attachment_data/file/416780/HBN_08-02.pdf (Last accessed 2.9.2021).

National Institute for Health and Care Excellence (NICE) (2018). Dementia: assessment, management and support for people living with dementia and their carers. https://www.nice.org.uk/guidance/ng97/resources/dementia-assessment-management-and-support-for-people-living-with-dementia-and-their-carers-pdf-1837760199109 (Last accessed 2.9.2021).

National Institute for Health and Care Excellence (NICE) (2019). *Dementia.* https://www.nice.org.uk/guidance/qs184/chapter/Quality-statement-2-Diagnosis (Last accessed 2.9.2021).

NHS England (2016). *The Well Pathway for Dementia.* https://www.england.nhs.uk/mentalhealth/wp-content/uploads/sites/29/2016/03/dementia-well-pathway.pdf (Last accessed 2.9.2021).

NHS UK (2018). *Help and support for people with dementia.* https://www.nhs.uk/conditions/dementia/help-and-support/ (Last accessed 2.9.2021).

NHS UK (2020a). *About dementia.* https://www.nhs.uk/conditions/dementia/about/ (Last accessed 2.9.2021).

NHS UK (2020b). *Can dementia be prevented?* https://www.nhs.uk/conditions/dementia/dementia-prevention/ (Last accessed 2.9.2021).

Patient.info website (2021). *Screening for cognitive impairment.* https://patient.info/doctor/screening-for-cognitive-impairment (Last accessed 2.9.2021).

Public Health England (PHE) (2018). *Dementia: applying All Our Health.* https://www.gov.uk/government/publications/dementia-applying-all-our-health/dementia-applying-all-our-health (Last accessed 2.9.2021).

Wittenberg, R., Hu, B., Barraza-Araiza, L. *et al.* (2019). *Projections of older people with dementia and costs of dementia care in the United Kingdom, 2019–2040.* London: Care Policy and Evaluation Centre, London School of Economics and Political Science (Last accessed 2.9.2021).

CHAPTER 7

Addiction

Learning outcomes

By the end of this chapter the reader will:

- Understand what is meant by addiction
- Be aware of different types of addiction
- Know how to screen for an addiction to alcohol and recognise an addiction to substances
- Recognise when a person may be addicted to a behaviour
- Be aware of the management options in primary care for people with an addiction

Introduction

Addiction means having no control over doing, taking, or using something, to the point where it could be harmful (NHS UK 2021). The substance or behaviour can create a feeling that is both physically and psychologically pleasurable. There are usually four stages of addiction, starting with experimentation, moving on to social or regular, then problem or risk, and lastly dependency. The person with an addiction will often need to use more of the substance or engage in the behaviour for longer to achieve the same feeling again. The long-term adverse outcomes can be physical, psychological, social and economic.

A person's genetic make-up can affect how susceptible they are to developing an addiction (Foll, Gallo, *et al.* 2009). It is estimated that 40–60% of a person's risk of developing addiction is based on genetics (Bevilacqua & Goldman 2009). Environment and culture also play a part in how a person responds to a substance or behaviour. People who have a disrupted social support system or have had traumatic experiences that affect their coping abilities are more susceptible (National Institute on Drug Abuse 2020).

Types of addiction

Addiction can be to a particular substance or to carrying out a certain behaviour.

Addiction to substances

The American Psychiatric Association (2017) explains that addiction is a brain disease which is manifested by compulsive substance use despite harmful consequences. People focus on using the substance to the point where it takes over their life, and they keep using it even when they know it will cause problems.

People can become addicted to substances including drugs, alcohol and nicotine (APA 2013). Caffeine use disorder is also recognised by the American Psychiatric Association in their diagnostic manual but it is listed under conditions requiring further research.

Drugs

The 2015 to 2016 Crime Survey for England and Wales (Home Office 2016) showed that 8% of people aged 16 to 59 had taken an illegal drug or used a substance unlawfully in the previous year, and 4% had taken one in the past month. Around 3% were defined as frequent drug users (having taken an illegal drug or used a substance unlawfully more than once a month, on average, in the past year). Figures were higher among young adults aged 16 to 24 (18% in the past year and 9% in the past month and 5% frequent).

Drugs commonly misused include marijuana, hallucinogens (e.g. LSD), dissociative drugs (e.g. PCP), opioid painkillers (e.g., codeine and oxycodone, heroin), sedatives, hypnotics and anxiolytics (medicines for anxiety such as tranquilisers), cocaine, methamphetamine and other stimulants (APA 2013). Inhalants, such as paint thinners and glue, are also addictive.

The non-medical use of drugs may result in serious clinical effects with potential life-threatening complications, drug-seeking behaviour, dependence, and related withdrawal symptoms (Chiappini & Schifano 2020).

According to the National Institute on Drug Abuse (2020), the groups of people at risk of drug misuse are those who:
- Have mental health problems
- Are being sexually exploited or sexually assaulted
- Are involved in commercial sex work
- Are lesbian, gay, bisexual or transgender
- Are not in employment, education or training
- Are considered homeless
- Attend nightclubs and festivals
- Are known to use drugs occasionally or recreationally.

Children and young people at risk are those who:
- Have carers or families who use drugs
- Are looked after or are care leavers
- Are in contact with young offender teams but not in secure environments (e.g. prisons and young offender institutions)
- Are excluded from school or who truant regularly.

Alcohol

To keep health risks from alcohol low, the UK Chief Medical Officers' (CMO) low-risk drinking guidelines advise it is safest for men and women not to drink more than 14 units a week on a regular basis, to limit the amount consumed on any single occasion, have several drink-free days each week, and spread consumption over three or more days if drinking as much as 14 units a week (DoH 2016).

In England and Scotland, 24% of adults regularly drink over these low-risk guidelines (PHE 2016), and 27% of drinkers in the UK binge-drink (over 8 units for men and over 6 units for women) on their heaviest drinking days (ONS 2018). In the UK in 2018 there were 7,551 alcohol-specific deaths (ONS 2019). It is estimated that in 2017/18 there were 586,779 dependent drinkers in England but only 18% of these were accessing treatment (PHE 2019).

In the UK, alcohol misuse is the greatest risk factor for death, ill-health and disability in people aged 15 to 49 years and the fifth highest risk factor for all ages (DoH 2016). Alcohol misuse is associated with disease and injuries, including infectious disease, cancer, diabetes, neuropsychiatric disease, cardiovascular disease, liver and pancreas disease and unintentional and intentional injury (Rehm 2011).

There is no single identified cause that leads to the development of alcoholism but there are significant risk factors. These include:

- Having a close family member with a diagnosis of a substance use disorder (genetic component or learnt behaviour or both)
- A diagnosis of mental illness
- An experience of trauma and/or stress
- Subclinical levels of stress
- A lack of family supervision or involvement
- Peer pressure
- Starting to drink at an early age
- Being male
- Living in an environment where alcohol use is acceptable and considered to be a standard approach to dealing with stress.

Nicotine

A survey by the Office for National statistics (2020) found that in the year 2019 in the UK:

- 14.1% of people aged 18 and above smoked cigarettes, compared with 14.7% in 2018
- 15.9% of men smoked, compared with 12.5% of women
- Those aged 25 to 34 had the highest proportion of current smokers (19.0%)
- 23.4% of people in routine and manual occupations smoked, compared to 9.3% of people in managerial and professional occupations
- 52.7% of people aged 16 and above, who currently smoked, wanted to quit.

Caffeine

Caffeine is the common name for 1,3,7-trimethylxanthine. It acts as a central nervous system stimulant. Intake of low to moderate doses of caffeine is generally safe, but clinical studies show that some caffeine users become dependent on the drug and are unable to reduce their consumption, despite knowledge of health problems associated with continued use (Meredith, Juliano, *et al.* 2013).

Depending on how much caffeine is taken and how it affects them, within 30 minutes after consuming it and for up to six hours, the person may feel: more alert and active, restless, excited, dizzy, anxious, irritable, thirsty, a need to urinate, heart pounding, unable to concentrate; they may also experience headache and stomach pains (Cappelletti, Piacentino, *et al.* 2015).

Caffeine withdrawal syndrome occurs when people skip a dose of caffeine and experience headaches, fatigue, depression, and trouble concentrating (APA 2013); so, they might continue to use caffeine to avoid these symptoms. It is unlikely that a toxic amount of caffeine can be consumed from caffeinated beverages alone but there have been deaths caused by ventricular fibrillation due to people consuming caffeine in tablet or powder form (Cappelletti, Piacentino, *et al.* 2018).

Addiction to a behaviour

People can become addicted to any behaviour that produces a strong reward (Addictions UK 2020) and this can result in problems in many areas of their lives (Alavi, Ferdosi, *et al.* 2012). The addictions can relate to any normal behaviour, such as social networking, work, shopping or exercise. Due to a lack of empirical evidence, these do not have a psychiatric diagnosis (APA 2013).

It is important to note that frequently indulging in some of these behaviours does not necessarily mean the person has an addiction (Erikson 2018). Gambling is recognised as a psychiatric condition; and internet gaming disorder (not general internet use or social media) is regarded by the American Psychiatric Association as requiring further research.

Gambling

A person with gambling disorder repeats problematic gambling behaviour that causes significant problems or distress. The condition is also referred to as gambling addiction or compulsive gambling. According to the American Psychiatric Association's guidance (2013), a diagnosis of gambling disorder requires at least four of the following during the past year:

1. A need to gamble with an increasing amount of money to achieve the desired excitement
2. Feeling restless or irritable when trying to cut down or stop gambling
3. Repeated unsuccessful efforts to control, reduce or stop gambling
4. Frequent thoughts about gambling (such as reliving past gambling experiences, planning the next gambling venture, thinking of ways to get money to gamble)
5. Often gambling when feeling distressed
6. After losing money gambling, often returning to 'get even' (referred to as 'chasing' one's losses)

7. Lying to conceal gambling activity
8. Jeopardising or losing a significant relationship, job or educational/career opportunity because of gambling
9. Relying on others to help with money problems caused by gambling.

A report on gambling in Great Britain (Gambling Commission 2017) stated that problem gambling prevalence in 2015 was 0.8%, with men being more likely than women to be classified as problem gamblers (1.5% and 0.2% respectively). The authors of this report explain that online gambling is on the increase, and it tends to occur alongside mental health problems and there are higher rates of suicide amongst problem gamblers.

Gaming disorder

The American Psychiatric Association (2013) identifies gaming disorder as requiring further research, but in 2019 the World Health Organization (2019) classified it as a mental health condition. WHO defines gaming disorder as a pattern of persistent or recurrent gaming behaviour so severe that it takes precedence over other life interests. The symptoms of gaming disorder include diminished control over gaming, increased priority given to gaming, and continuation or intensification of gaming despite negative consequences, such as negative impact on relationships, social life, studying and work life or increasing financial costs.

Gaming disorder may also be referred to as gaming addiction or video game addiction (VGA). There is little research on the prevalence of gaming disorder, but a study carried out in four countries including the UK which surveyed 19,000 men and women, found that over half of the participants said they had played internet games recently (Przybylski, Weinstein & Murayama 2017). Of these, between 1% and 0.5% said they had feelings of significant distress about being unable to curb their play.

Social networking site addiction

Social networking has become a regular behaviour for many people. They log onto social networking sites such as Facebook to interact. Research has indicated that more than 350 million people globally meet the clinical definition of an addiction because of their Facebook habits (Gaille 2017), and Facebook addiction is only one example of social networking site addiction (Kuss & Griffiths 2017).

Studies have shown that addiction to Facebook is positively associated with depression, anxiety, and insomnia (Hou, Xion, et al. 2019). Social networking site addiction may include a fear of missing out, and anxiety about not having a working mobile phone (Kuss & Griffiths 2017). A study of social networking site addiction showed that it was strongly associated with internet addiction (Yu, Wu, et al. 2016). It has been claimed that over-reliance on technology has led to an impoverishment of social skills and that people have come to be described as 'alone together', always connected via technology, but in fact isolated (Turkle 2013, 2015).

Work addiction

Experts in the field of work addiction agree that it is a problematic behaviour that needs more research (Atroszko, Demetrovics & Griffiths 2019). They have put forward a tentative general definition of work addiction which states that it is:

> …characterized by a compulsion to work and preoccupation with work activities leading to a significant harm and distress of a functionally impairing nature to the individual and/or other significantly relevant relationships (friends and family). The behaviour is characterized by the loss of control over the working activity and persists over a significant period of time. This problematic work-related behaviour can have varying intensity from mild to severe.

As agreement still needs to be reached on the definition of work addiction, it is difficult to understand how many people are affected by it. Some estimates are as high as 15%–25% among employed individuals (Griffiths, Demetrovics & Atroszko 2018).

Shopping addiction

Shopping addiction is referred to by some experts in the field as buying-shopping disorder or BSD (Müller, Brand, *et al.* 2019). People with this condition are preoccupied with buying things, and they cannot control their spending despite negative consequences, such as debt, and family and work conflicts (Müller, Mitchell, *et al.* 2015).

It has been defined as 'being overly concerned about shopping, driven by an uncontrollable shopping motivation, and to investing so much time and effort into shopping that it impairs other important life areas' (Andreassen, Griffiths, *et al.* 2015). People who are addicted to shopping often have poor self-esteem and marked distress or have a common mental disorder (Murali, Ray & Shaffiullha 2012). A meta-analysis of 40 studies reporting 49 prevalence estimates from 16 countries (n = 32,000) indicated an estimated point prevalence of BSD of 5% (Maraz, Griffiths & Demetrovics 2016).

Exercise addiction

Exercise is generally beneficial for mental health and can help people manage mild depression or severe anxiety. However, over-exercising can have a negative impact. People who are primarily addicted to exercise feel they must exercise, and the amount they do can become excessive (Szabo, Griffiths, *et al.* 2015). It is not the same as the extreme exercise observed in people with eating disorders where the exercise is a way to control weight.

Exercise addiction is not officially classified as a mental health disorder, but it can have similar negative effects on emotional and social health as other addictions (Hausenblas, Schreiber & Smoliga 2017). Using a fitness tracker can feed into exercise addiction and sharing data on social media means that exercising becomes public and competitive.

An observational study showed that symptoms of exercise addiction ranged from 0.3% to 0.5% in the general population (Mónok, Berczik, *et al.* 2012), and in a study of people who regularly exercised it varied between 1.9% and 3.2% (Griffiths, Urbán, *et al.* 2015).

Management options in primary care

Healthcare professionals can advise and support people to manage their addictions.

Drugs

National guidance for drug misuse prevention places a responsibility on healthcare professionals in primary care to use routine appointments to assess whether someone is vulnerable to drug misuse (NICE 2017). The guidance states that these people include those: in multiple groups at risk; whose personal circumstances put them at increased risk; who may already be using drugs on an occasional basis; who may already be regularly excessively consuming another substance, such as alcohol; and young people aged 10 to 18 (or aged up to 25 with special educational needs or a disability).

It can be difficult to identify drug misuse, as people will often deny that they have a problem, and it is rare for primary care practitioners to proactively screen for substance use. Usually, drug misuse is uncovered when the person presents at the practice in a distressed state requesting help. They may ask for:

- A prescription for drugs
- Help to withdraw or stabilise their drug use
- Treatment for the physical complications of drug use, such as abscesses
- Medical acknowledgement of a drug problem because of debt or prosecution.

Diagnosis of a substance misuse disorder should be based on a comprehensive history. Some useful questions include:

- Has using drugs resulted in:
  - o Physical injury or illness?
  - o Emotional distress or mental illness?
  - o Social problems such as breakdown of relationships or job loss?
- How often do you take drugs?
- Do you crave drugs?
- Are you unable to stop using drugs?
- Do the drugs you take no longer have the effect they used to?
- Do you have withdrawal symptoms when you stop taking drugs (e.g. increased heart rate, sweating, tremors)?
- What are your reasons for attending the practice today?
- Have you got a history of physical or mental illness?

Examination may include:

- Checking for physical symptoms, e.g. nausea, constipation, drowsiness
- Screening for depression using the PHQ-9
- Laboratory investigations: full blood count, liver function test, hepatitis B and C screen, urine drug screen.

People who need treatment for drug addiction are entitled to NHS care in the same way as anyone else who has a health problem (NHS UK 2021). Adults identified should be offered clear information on drugs and their effects, advice and feedback on any existing drug use, and information on local services and where to find further advice and support. Children and young people who are assessed as vulnerable to drug misuse should be offered skills training where it is commissioned.

The Frank website (2021) lists local drug treatment services and provides honest information about drugs. When a person is supported by a drug treatment service, they are usually given a keyworker to support them throughout their treatment. The treatment will depend on the person's personal circumstances and what they are addicted to, and may include:

- Talking therapies
- Medication
- Detoxification (detox)
- Self-help, such as attending support groups like Narcotics Anonymous
- Testing and treatment for hepatitis or HIV.

Alcohol

It is rare for a person to attend primary care and state that they have a drink problem. Most will either deny or be unaware of the seriousness of their alcohol problem, so it is important for healthcare professionals to be proactive in checking how much alcohol people are drinking. Some may present with physical symptoms which are complications of alcohol use, such as an ulcer, gastritis, liver disease or accidental injury. Low mood, poor memory or concentration, and insomnia, may also be a sign that the person has a problem with alcohol.

Alcohol misuse may be noticed when the person has tried to cut down or stop drinking alcohol and experiences withdrawal symptoms that may include sweating and tremors. Some people drink to self-medicate an underlying mental health problem, particularly depression. Screening for alcohol use can be carried out by using the alcohol use disorders identification test for primary care (AUDIT-PC 2021). This is the short version of the full 10-question AUDIT and is very quick to administer. It will indicate whether an individual is potentially drinking at increasing or higher risk levels but cannot determine the type of intervention required and does not indicate alcohol dependence. It can be downloaded from the government's website.

AUDIT-PC

Questions	Scoring system					Your score
	1	**2**	**3**	**4**	**5**	
How often do you have a drink containing alcohol?	Never	Monthly or less	2–4 times per month	2–3 times per week	4+ times per week	
How many units of alcohol do you drink on a typical day when you are drinking?	1–2	3–4	5–6	7–9	10+	
How often during the last year have you found that you were not able to stop drinking once you had started?	Never	Less than monthly	Monthly	Weekly	Daily or almost daily	
How often during the last year have you failed to do what was normally expected from you because of your drinking?	Never	Less than monthly	Monthly	Weekly	Daily or almost daily	
Has a relative or friend, doctor or other health worker been concerned about your drinking or suggested that you cut down?	No		Yes, but not in the last year		Yes, during the last year	

A total score of 5 or more indicates increasing or higher risk drinking and is classed as AUDIT-PC positive. In these cases, the full test should be used. The remaining questions are in the table below.

Remaining questions

Questions	Scoring system					Your score
	0	**1**	**2**	**3**	**4**	
How often have you had 6 or more units if female, or 8 or more if male, on a single occasion in the last year?	Never	Less than monthly	Monthly	Weekly	Daily or almost daily	
How often during the last year have you needed an alcoholic drink in the morning to get yourself going after a heavy drinking session?	Never	Less than monthly	Monthly	Weekly	Daily or almost daily	

How often during the last year have you had a feeling of guilt or remorse after drinking?	Never	Less than monthly	Monthly	Weekly	Daily or almost daily	
How often during the last year have you been unable to remember what happened the night before because you had been drinking?	Never	Less than monthly	Monthly	Weekly	Daily or almost daily	
Has a relative or friend, doctor or other health worker been concerned about your drinking or suggested that you cut down?	No		Yes, but not in the last year		Yes, during the last year	

A score of 0–7 indicates lower risk, 8–15 increasing risk, 16–19 higher risk, and 20 or more is possible dependence. In those people identified as misusing or being dependent on alcohol, it is worth considering screening for depression.

Helping a person to reduce or stop alcohol is usually more successful with specialist support. Many areas have their own local centre which focuses on helping people with alcohol problems. Entering the name of the town or postcode into the Frank website (2021) will enable you to access this information: https://www.talktofrank.com/get-help/find-support-near-you

Reducing alcohol can precipitate an acute loss of thiamine (vitamin B1) stores in people who may already be chronically thiamine deficient. Thiamine deficiency is associated with Wernicke-Korsakoff syndrome (alcoholic brain disease) and beriberi (neurological symptoms, cardiovascular abnormalities and oedema). A thiamine preparation to prevent these conditions should be considered.

Some people will not be willing to stop drinking. In these cases, the healthcare professional should work towards reducing harm by encouraging the person to cut down the amount they drink and provide information about the detrimental effects of drinking.

Nicotine

National guidance recommends that primary care health practitioners deliver 'Very Brief Advice' or 'VBA' to people who smoke (NICE 2018). It takes less than 30 seconds and uses the 'AAA' framework (National Centre for Smoking Cessation and Training 2014) where practitioners:

- Ask about smoking to establish the person's smoking status and record this
- Advise on how they can stop smoking
- Act by offering help to support them to quit, including referring people to stop smoking services (SSS) or prescribing pharmacotherapy with brief advice.

A survey on behalf of Cancer Research (Rosenberg, Crawford, *et al.* 2019) found that, though 84% of healthcare professionals in primary care ask about smoking and 87% offer advice on how to quit, only 64% take action to support their patients to quit. They suggest that, to follow national guidance, primary care health practitioners need to complete training in VBA and be aware of treatment options available to people in their local area, including prescribing pharmacotherapy or referral to specialist stop smoking services in their practice or community. They also advocate the use of e-cigarettes as an aid to stop smoking, recommending that they be used alongside behavioural support.

When a person wants to stop smoking, NICE (2018) recommends that health and social care workers in primary and community settings should:

- Refer people who want to stop smoking to local stop smoking support.
- Discuss how to stop smoking with people who want to quit (see table below).
- Set out the pharmacotherapy and behavioural options: offer behavioural support (individual and group); bupropion; nicotine replacement therapy (NRT) – short and long acting; varenicline; and very brief advice. Take into consideration their previous use of stop smoking aids, and any adverse effects and contraindications for the different pharmacotherapies.
- Explain that a combination of varenicline and behavioural support or a combination of short-acting and long-acting NRT are likely to be most effective.
- If people opt out of a referral to local stop smoking support, refer them to a professional who can offer pharmacotherapy and Very Brief Advice.
- Agree the approach to stopping smoking that best suits the person's preferences and review this approach at future visits.

Tips for stopping smoking
<ul><li>List your reasons to stop.</li><li>Tell people you are stopping.</li><li>If you have tried to stop before, remember what worked.</li><li>Use stop smoking aids.</li><li>Have a plan if you are tempted to smoke.</li><li>List your smoking triggers and how to avoid them.</li><li>Keep cravings at bay by keeping busy.</li><li>Exercise away the urge.</li><li>Join the Smokefree Quit Smoking Facebook group for support and advice: https://www.facebook.com/groups/707621863012993/?source_id=162994267161135</li></ul>

Adapted from NHS (2021).

Caffeine

As it is difficult know exactly how much caffeine they consume, people should be advised to put a limit on the total amount of caffeinated products they eat and drink and be aware that decaffeinated products still contain a small amount of caffeine. They can also choose products with lower caffeine contents. Chapter 2 (p. 28) lists the caffeine content of many drinks and chocolate-containing products.

There are no formal guidelines to help people reduce their caffeine intake, but strategies that are effective in stopping other problem behaviours (such as smoking, drinking alcohol or overeating) may help with caffeine reduction (see Chapter 2). These include looking out for triggers that spur caffeine use and asking friends to help them reach their goal (Budney, Lee & Juliano 2015). One study showed that a brief one-session manualised intervention with follow-up was efficacious at reducing caffeine consumption (Evatt, Juliano & Griffiths 2016). The intervention included a session provided by a trained counsellor along with a take-home booklet (Evatt, Juliano & Griffiths 2016). After the session, participants completed daily diaries of caffeine consumption for five weeks and returned for follow-up assessments.

Gambling

The charity GambleAware (2020) reports that the number of people receiving help for gambling disorder is currently low (only 1–2%) and advises that if there was more awareness of the support that is available for gambling, people would be more motivated to seek treatment. They have campaigned for people in Great Britain with gambling disorder to contact the National Gambling Treatment Service website to access free care. This service is made up of a network of NHS trusts and voluntary sector organisations. They provide telephone, online, and face-to-face treatment for individuals and groups.

GambleAware (2020) advise healthcare professionals in primary care to ask people who present with issues such as depression, anxiety, loneliness, and financial difficulties a simple question to try to identify whether they have gambling disorder. They suggest asking:

'In the last 12 months, have you bet more than you can really afford to lose? Or has this happened to someone close to you?'

If the person responds positively, they should be advised to contact the National Gambling Treatment Service by ringing their helpline **(0808 8020 133)** or visiting BeGambleAware (2021), a website where they can chat live online. This service is available 24 hours a day, seven days a week. The charity Gamcare (2021) also provides information and support for people wanting to stop gambling, including a helpline and online forum.

Gaming disorder

The symptoms of gaming disorder can be similar to the symptoms of mental illnesses including depression (Freeman 2008). Therefore, healthcare professionals may consider whether gaming disorder has a role in the person's current condition. To assess an individual for gaming disorder, Chen, Oliffe and Kelly (2018) suggest using nine open-ended questions based on the diagnostic criteria proposed by the

American Psychiatric Association (2013). Healthcare professionals can ask the following questions based on the diagnostic criteria:

- How much time do you spend thinking about gaming?
- How do you feel when you cannot play?
- Do you find that you need to spend more and more time playing to feel good?
- Do you feel unable to quit or even play less?
- Do you not want to do other things that you used to like doing?
- Are you having problems at work, school or home because of your gaming?
- Are you still playing despite these problems?
- Are you lying to people close to you about how much time you spend playing?
- Are you using gaming to ease bad moods and feelings?

Healthcare professionals working in primary care in England and Wales can refer people aged 13 and over to the National Centre for Gaming Disorders. The service is led by a consultant psychiatrist and staffed by psychologists and family therapists who assess and treat the needs of problem gamers as well as their family members or carers (NHS Central and North West London 2021).

Social networking

There is currently no specific national clinical guidance for recognising and treating social networking site addiction, but experts in psychology recommend six questions to ask a person who may be addicted to social media (Andreassen 2015):

1. Do you spend a lot of time when you are not online thinking about social media or planning to use social media?
2. Do you feel urges to use social media more and more over time?
3. Do you use social media to forget about personal problems?
4. Do you often try to reduce your use of social media, without success?
5. Do you become restless or troubled if you are unable to use social media?
6. Do you use social media so much that it has had a negative impact on your job, relationship or studies?

If a few of the questions are answered positively, they advise that the person is probably a typical, habitual social media user who may benefit from reducing the amount of time spent on social media. This can be achieved through a few basic steps such as turning off the sound function on their phone, only allowing themselves to check their phone every hour or so, and dedicating periods in the day as self-imposed no-screen time. However, if they answer 'yes' to most or all the questions, they may have, or be developing, an actual addiction to using social media.

The problems associated with social networking site addiction can be treated using self-help methods, relaxation exercises, cognitive behavioural therapy techniques, and medications such as antidepressants (Andreassen 2015).

Work addiction

There is currently no specific national clinical guidance for recognising and treating work addiction. The Bergen Work Addiction Scale uses seven basic criteria to identify work addiction, where all items are scored on the following scale: 1 (never), 2 (rarely), 3 (sometimes), 4 (often) and 5 (always):

1. You think of how you can free up more time to work.
2. You spend much more time working than initially intended.
3. You work in order to reduce feelings of guilt, anxiety, helplessness and depression.
4. You have been told by others to cut down on work without listening to them.
5. You become stressed if you are prohibited from working.
6. You prioritise work over hobbies, leisure activities and exercise.
7. You work so much it has negatively influenced your health.

A score of 4 or 5 on four or more of these criteria suggests the person may be experiencing work addiction (Andreassen *et al.* 2012):

The problems associated with work addiction may be treated using self-help methods, relaxation exercises, and cognitive behavioural therapy techniques.

Shopping addiction

There is currently no specific national clinical guidance for recognising and treating shopping addiction. The Bergen Shopping Addiction Scale uses seven basic criteria to identify shopping addiction (Andreassen, Griffiths, *et al.* 2015). All the items are scored on the following scale: (0) completely disagree, (1) disagree, (2) neither disagree nor agree, (3) agree, and (4) completely agree:

1. You think about shopping/buying things all the time.
2. You shop/buy things in order to change your mood.
3. You shop/buy so much that it negatively affects your daily obligations (e.g., school and work).
4. You feel you have to shop/buy more and more to obtain the same satisfaction as before.
5. You have decided to shop/buy less but have not been able to do so.
6. You feel bad if, for some reason, you are prevented from shopping/buying things.
7. You shop/buy so much that it has impaired your well-being.

A score of 'agree' or 'completely agree' on at least four of the seven items may suggest that the person is addicted to shopping.

Treatment for shopping addiction usually involves practical solutions such as consolidation of debt and organising a third party to control finances, and healthier ways to manage negative feelings such as cognitive behavioural therapy. If the shopping addiction is driven by anxiety or depression, then anti-depressant medication may be prescribed. There are several support groups available for people with a shopping addiction, including Shopaholics Anonymous (https://www.facebook.com/Shopaholics-Anonymous-UK-254923888369982/), Spenders Anonymous (http://www.spenders.org/) and Debtors Anonymous (https://debtorsanonymous.org.uk/).

Exercise addiction

There is currently no specific national clinical guidance for recognising and treating exercise addiction. Griffiths, Szabo & Terry (2005) developed a screening tool for healthcare providers which comprises six criteria. The questions are scored as: (1) strongly disagree, (2) disagree, (3) neither agree nor disagree, (4) agree, (5) strongly agree:

1. Exercise is the most important thing in my life.
2. Conflicts have arisen between me and my family and/or my partner about the amount of exercise I do.
3. I use exercise as a way of changing my mood.
4. Over time I have increased the amount of exercise I do in a day.
5. If I have to miss an exercise session, I feel moody and irritable.
6. If I cut down the amount of exercise I do, and then start again, I always end up exercising as often as I did before.

A total score ≥24 (out of 30) indicates that the person is at risk for exercise addiction and should be referred to an appropriate specialist. A score of 13–23 indicates a potentially symptomatic person and a score of 0–12 indicates no problems.

Cognitive behavioural therapy is recommended to restructure maladaptive beliefs about exercise and manage mood disturbances (Weinstein & Weinstein 2014). It may help the person to work with fitness professionals to create an appropriate training routine and learn to differentiate between appropriate versus excessive training and healthy versus unhealthy motivators, such as comparison with others (Hausenblas, Schreiber & Smoliga 2017).

Summary

Addiction involves doing, taking or using something which may result in physical, psychological, social and economic long-term adverse outcomes. Healthcare professionals working in primary care can help people recognise they have an addiction and support them to get the most appropriate treatment and support.

> ## Vignette
>
> Vincent is 68 years old and has come for his NHS health check. He explains that since retiring he has taken up running to keep fit and jokes that it is also to stay out of his wife's way. He has hurt his knee but says that is not stopping him going out twice a day, to run for an hour or more, as it is something he really needs to do. The healthcare professional notices that he looks tired and very thin.
>
> How should the healthcare professional explore the possibility of exercise addiction?

Reflective questions

- How does your practice help people with an addiction? Is there a protocol in place?
- Think about a person who came to see you with a problem that may have been related to an addiction. Did you explore the possibility? If not, what would you do differently next time?
- How would you engage with a person who you feel has an addiction, but they say that their behaviour is normal for them?

References

Addictions UK (2020). *Addictive Behaviour.* https://addictionsuk.com/addictive-behaviour/ (Last accessed 4.9.2021).

Alavi, S., Ferdosi, M., Jannatifard, F. *et al.* (2012). Behavioral addiction versus substance addiction: correspondence of psychiatric and psychological views. *International Journal of Preventive Medicine.* **3** (4), 290–294.

American Psychiatric Association (APA) (2013). *The Diagnostic and Statistical Manual of Mental Disorders.* 5th edn. Arlington VA: APA.

American Psychiatric Association (APA) (2017). *What is addiction?* https://www.psychiatry.org/patients-families/addiction/what-is-addiction (Last accessed 4.9.2021).

Andreassen, C. (2015). Online social network site addiction: a comprehensive review. *Current Addiction Reports.* **2**, 175–184.

Andreassen, C., Billieux, J., Griffiths, M. *et al.* (2016). The relationship between addictive use of social media and video games and symptoms of psychiatric disorders: A large-scale cross-sectional study. *Psychology of Addictive Behaviours.* **30** (2), 252–262.

Andreassen, C., Griffiths., M, Hetland., J. *et al.* (2012). Development of a work addiction scale. *Scandinavian Journal of Psychology.* **53** (3), 265–272.

Andreassen, C., Griffiths, M., Hetland, J. *et al.* (2014). The prevalence of workaholism: a survey study in a nationally representative sample of Norwegian employees. *PLoS ONE* 9:e102446 10.1371/journal.pone.0102446

Andreassen, C., Griffiths, M., Pallesen, S. *et al.* (2015). The Bergen Shopping Addiction Scale: reliability and validity of a brief screening test. *Frontiers in Psychology.* **17** (6), 1374.

Atroszko, P.A., Demetrovics, Z., & Griffiths, M.D. (2019). Beyond the myths about work addiction: Toward a consensus on definition and trajectories for future studies on problematic overworking. *Journal of Behavioral Addictions.* **8** (1), 7–15. https://doi.org/10.1556/2006.8.2019.11 (Last accessed 4.9.2021).

AUDIT-PC (2021). https://assets.publishing.service.gov.uk/government/uploads/system/uploads/attachment_data/file/684824/Alcohol_use_disorders_identification_test_for_primary_care__AUDIT_PC_.pdf (Last accessed 4.9.2021).

BeGambleAware/The National Gambling Treatment Service (2021). https://www.begambleaware.org/ngts (Last accessed 4.9.2021).

Bevilacqua, L. & Goldman, D. (2009). Genes and addictions. *Clinical Pharmacology and Therapeutics.* **85** (4), 359–361.

Budney, A., Lee, D. & Juliano, L. (2015). Evaluating the validity of caffeine use disorder. *Current Psychiatry Reports.* **17** (9).

Cappelletti, S., Piacentino, D., Sani, G. *et al.* (2015). Caffeine: Cognitive and physical performance enhancer or psychoactive drug? *Current Neuropharmacology.* **13**, 71–88.

Cappelletti, S., Piacentino, D., Fineschi, V. *et al.* (2018). Caffeine-related deaths: Manner of deaths and categories at risk. *Nutrients.* **10** (5), 611.

Chen, K., Oliffe, J. & Kelly, M. (2018). Internet gaming disorder: An emergent health issue for men. *American Journal of Men's Health.* **12** (4), 1151–1159.

Chiappini, S. & Schifano, F. (2020). What about 'pharming'? Issues regarding the misuse of prescription and over-the-counter drugs. *Brain Science.* **10** (10), 736.

Department of Health (DoH) (2016). UK Chief Medical Officers' Low Risk Drinking Guidelines. London: DoH.

Erikson, C. (2018). *The Science of Addiction.* 2nd revised edn. London: Norton Professional Books.

Evatt, D., Juliano, L. & Griffiths, R. (2016). A brief manualized treatment for problematic caffeine use: A randomized control trial. *Journal of Consulting and Clinical Psychology.* **84** (2), 113–121.

Foll, B., Gallo, A., Strat, Y. *et al.* (2009). Genetics of dopamine receptors and drug addiction: a comprehensive review. *Behavioural Pharmacology.* **20** (1), 1–17.

Frank website (2021). https://www.talktofrank.com (Last accessed 4.9.2021).

Freeman, C. (2008). Internet gaming addiction. *The Journal for Nurse Practitioners.* **4** (1), 42–47.

Gaille, B. (2017). *43 remarkable Facebook addiction statistics.* https://brandongaille.com/42-remarkable-facebook-addiction-statistics/ (Last accessed 4.9.2021).

GambleAware (2020). *National Gambling Treatment Service Campaign*. https://www.begambleaware.org/national-gambling-treatment-service-campaign (Last accessed 4.9.2021).

Gambling Commission (2017). *Gambling behaviour in Great Britain in 2015*. http://www.gamblingcommission.gov.uk/PDF/survey-data/Gambling-behaviour-in-Great-Britain-2015.pdf (Last accessed 4.9.2021).

GamCare (2021). https://www.gamcare.org.uk/ (Last accessed 4.9.2021).

Griffiths, M., Demetrovics, Z. & Atroszko, P. (2018). Ten myths about work addiction. *Journal of Behavioral Addictions*. **7** (4), 845–857.

Griffiths, M., Szabo, A. & Terry, A. (2005). The exercise addiction inventory: a quick and easy screening tool for health practitioners. *British Journal of Sports Medicine*. **357**, e30.

Griffiths, M., Urbán, R., Demetrovics, Z. *et al.* (2015). A cross-cultural re-evaluation of the Exercise Addiction Inventory (EAI) in five countries. *Sports Medicine Open*. **357**, 5.

Hausenblas, H., Schreiber, K. & Smoliga, J. (2017). Addiction to exercise. *British Medical Journal*. **357**.

Home Office (2016). Drug misuse: findings from the 2015 to 2016 CSEW second edition. https://www.gov.uk/government/statistics/drug-misuse-findings-from-the-2015-to-2016-csew (Last accessed 4.9.2021).

Hou, Y., Xiong, D., Jiang, T. *et al.* (2019). Social media addiction: Its impact, mediation, and intervention. *Cyberpsychology*: *Journal of Psychosocial Research on Cyberspace*. **13** (1), Article 4.

Kuss, D. & Griffiths, M. (2017). Social networking sites and addiction: Ten lessons learned. *International Journal of Environmental Research and Public Health*. **14** (3), 311.

Maraz, A., Griffiths, M. & Demetrovics, Z. (2016). The prevalence of compulsive buying: a meta-analysis. *Addiction*. **111** (2016), 408–419.

Meredith, S., Juliano, L., Hughes, J. *et al.* (2013). Caffeine use disorder: A comprehensive review and research agenda. *Journal of Caffeine Research*. **3** (3), 114–130.

Mishra, A., Chaturvedi, P., Datta, S. *et al.* (2015). Harmful effects of nicotine. *Indian Journal of Medical and Paediatric Oncology*. **36** (1), 24–31.

Mónok, K., Berczik, K., Urbán, R., *et al.* (2012). Psychometric properties and concurrent validity of two exercise addiction measures: A population wide study. *Psychology of Sport and Exercise*. **357**, 739–746.

Müller, A., Brand, M., Claes, L. *et al.* (2019). Buying-shopping disorder—Is there enough evidence to support its inclusion in ICD-11? *CNS Spectrums*. **24** (4), 374–379.

Müller, A., Mitchell, J. & de Zwaan, M. (2015). Compulsive buying. *American Journal on Addictions*. **24** (2), 132–137.

Murali, V., Ray, R. & Shaffiullha, M. (2012). Shopping addiction. *Advances in Psychiatric Treatment*. **18** (4), 263–269.

National Centre for Smoking Cessation and Training (2014). *Very Brief Advice (VBA) on Smoking: the evidence*. https://www.ncsct.co.uk/publication_very-brief-advice.php (Last accessed 4.9.2021).

National Health Service (NHS) UK (2021). *Addiction: what is it?* https://www.nhs.uk/live-well/healthy-body/addiction-what-is-it/ (Last accessed 4.9.2021).

National Health Service (NHS) (2021). *Quit smoking*. https://www.nhs.uk/better-health/quit-smoking/?WT.mc_ID=JanQuitSmokingPPC&gclid=CMqDvIGjlu4CFclNGwodmmYlig (Last accessed 4.9.2021).

National Health Service (NHS) Central and North West London (2021). *National Centre for Gaming Disorders*. https://www.cnwl.nhs.uk/services/mental-health-services/addictions-and-substance-misuse/national-centre-behavioural-addictions/National-Centre-for-Gaming-Disorders (Last accessed 7.9.2021).

National Institute on Drug Abuse (NIDA) (2020). *Drug Misuse and Addiction*. https://www.drugabuse.gov/publications/drugs-brains-behavior-science-addiction/drug-misuse-addiction (Last accessed 4.9.2021).

National Institute for Health and Care Excellence (NICE) (2017). *Drug misuse prevention: targeted interventions*. https://www.nice.org.uk/guidance/ng64/resources/drug-misuse-prevention-targeted-interventions-pdf-1837573761733 (Last accessed 4.9.2021).

National Institute for Health and Care Excellence (NICE) (2018). *Stop smoking interventions and services*. https://www.nice.org.uk/guidance/ng92 (Last accessed 4.9.2021).

Office for National Statistics (ONS) (2018). *Adult drinking habits in Great Britain*. https://www.ons.gov.uk/peoplepopulationandcommunity/healthandsocialcare/drugusealcoholandsmoking/bulletins/opinionsandlifestylesurveyadultdrinkinghabitsingreatbritain/2017 (Last accessed 4.9.2021).

Office for National Statistics (ONS) (2019). *Alcohol-specific deaths in the UK: registered in 2018.* https://www.ons.gov.uk/peoplepopulationandcommunity/healthandsocialcare/causesofdeath/bulletins/alcoholrelateddeathsintheunitedkingdom/2018 (Last accessed 4.9.2021).

Office for National Statistics (ONS) (2020). *Adult smoking habits in the UK: 2019.* https://www.ons.gov.uk/peoplepopulationandcommunity/healthandsocialcare/healthandlifeexpectancies/bulletins/adultsmokinghabitsingreatbritain/2019 (Last accessed 7.9.2021).

Przybylski, A., Weinstein, N. & Murayama, K. (2017). Internet gaming disorder: Investigating the clinical relevance of a new phenomenon. *American Journal of Psychiatry.* **174** (3), 230–236.

Public Health England (PHE) (2016). *The Public Health Burden of Alcohol and the Effectiveness and Cost-Effectiveness of Alcohol Control Policies An evidence review.* London: PHE.

Public Health England (PHE) (2019). *Alcohol dependence prevalence in England.* London: PHE.

Rehm, J. (2011). The risks associated with alcohol use and alcoholism. *Alcohol Research & Health.* **34** (2), 135–143.

Rosenberg, G., Crawford, C., Bullock, S. *et al.* (2019). *Smoking Cessation in Primary Care: A cross-sectional survey of primary care health practitioners in the UK and the use of Very Brief Advice.* https://www.cancerresearchuk.org/sites/default/files/tobacco_pc_report_to_publish_-_full12.pdf (Last accessed 4.9.2021).

Szabo, A., Griffiths, M., de La Vega Marcos, R. *et al.* (2015). Methodological and conceptual limitations in exercise addiction research. *Yale Journal of Biological Medicine.* **357**, 303–308.

Turkle, S. (2013). *Alone Together. Why We Expect More from Technology and Less from Each Other.* Philadelphia: Basic Books.

Turkle, S. (2015). *Reclaiming Conversation: The Power of Talk in a Digital Age.* Penguin: New York.

Weinstein, A. & Weinstein, Y. (2014). Exercise addiction—diagnosis, bio-psychological mechanisms and treatment issues. *Current Pharmaceutical Design.* **357**, 4062–4069.

World Health Organization (WHO) (2019). International Classification of Diseases, 11th Revision: Mental, behavioural or neurodevelopmental disorders. https://icd.who.int/browse11/l-m/en#/http%3a%2f%2fid.who.int%2ficd%2fentity%2f334423054 (Last accessed 4.9.2021).

Yu, S., Wu, A. & Pesigan, I. (2016). Cognitive and psychosocial health risk factors of social networking addiction. *International Journal of Mental Health Addiction.* **14**, 550–564.

INDEX